FOOD
FOR
ATHLETES

FOOD FOR ATHLETES

Ann Lincoln

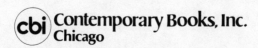
Contemporary Books, Inc.
Chicago

Library of Congress Cataloging in Publication Data

Lincoln, Ann.
    Food for athletes.

    Includes bibliographies and index.
    1. Athletes—Nutrition.   I. Title.
TX361.A8L48   1979   613.2′02′4796   78-27509
ISBN 0-8092-7503-1
ISBN 0-8092-7502-3 pbk.

Published by Contemporary Books, Inc.
180 North Michigan Avenue, Chicago, Illinois 60601
Manufactured in the United States of America
Library of Congress Catalog Card Number: 78-27509
International Standard Book Number: 0-8092-7503-1 (cloth)
                                    0-8092-7502-3 (paper)

Published simultaneously in Canada by
Beaverbooks
953 Dillingham Road
Pickering, Ontario L1W 1Z7
Canada

May the thoughts from this book
help you enjoy better health
for the rest of your life.

Contents

To my husband, Russell

Mission

This book is written for the athlete of any age and either sex; for the coach of any sport; and for parents concerned with feeding athletes.

It has been a privilege to be involved—as a teacher and as a parent—with school athletics. From years of study, observation, training, and practice has come the desire to translate nutritional material into layman's terms—from the viewpoint of a mother and with the pen of a home economist.

This book is about food and how it can assist the athlete in physical development, athletic training, and personal performance. Because material on nutrition in scientific journals often is complex, using unfamiliar terminology, it is my intention that this book be easy to read as well as accurate and encourage the reader to return again and again for further study and reference. Hopefully, it will be a prod to further study of food and the fascinating way our body uses it.

An important mission of this book is to promote the

realization of what a wonderful mechanism the human body is. One stands in awe of the workings of each minute cell, the pumping of the heart, the intricate functioning of the eyes and ears, to say nothing of the miracle of food digestion and its conversion to energy. How can one help but marvel at this wonderful human machine!

Although eating is a very personal thing, we should not expect "just any old food" to nourish us. A car owner services his automobile with meticulous care; shouldn't we exercise as much care in servicing our human machine! Usually, no replacement works as well as the original; no human organ is fully appreciated until it is too late.

I hope this book will be the inspiration for many athletes to dedicate their lives to pursuing good eating habits just as they develop exercise programs to last their entire lifetimes.

Ann Lincoln
Home Economist

Acknowledgment

I am grateful for the opportunity to share my interest in nutrition and my concern for reaching others with its message of importance for good health.

Nutrition is a complex subject and to one who is outside the profession, the terms are often unfamiliar and confusing. Trying to reduce nutrition information to more simple terms has been a labor of love—attempted in hopes this book could bring a timely message of guidance to good nutrition for athletes and non-athletes everywhere.

I would like to acknowledge a life-long debt to my mother. She realized the importance of food, especially vegetables, and served them creatively many years ago. Perhaps, as a result, good health has been my priceless legacy. Mother is well into her eighth decade and has been a constant encouragement, via letters, throughout this project.

Special thanks go to my husband for his continuing interest and also for his concern for detail and accuracy. Without all his assistance I could never have completed this demanding task.

Several members of the Foods and Nutrition Staff at Oregon State University have very kindly assisted with corrections and suggestions for improvements on segments of the material. The author is particularly endebted to Dr. Elizabeth Johnson, Dr. Elisabeth Yearick, and Prof. Jean Peters, of the University Food Staff, and to Ms. Carolyn Robb, Oregon State Nutrition Specialist, and to Mrs. Judy Burridge, Benton County (Oregon) Home Economics Extension Agent. The helpfulness of Prof. Georgene Barte of the University Food Staff is also much appreciated.

Personal thanks are given to Mrs. Jari Knudson, nutritionist, who kindly made suggestions and corrections. Helpful, also, in reading portions of material and making suggestions were Dr. Dale Thomas, head wrestling coach at Oregon State University, Dr. June McMurdo, health teacher, Mr. Doug Bashor, wrestling coach, Mr. Jerome Colonna, cross-country coach (the latter three are teachers in the Corvallis, Oregon, public school system); and thanks, too, to Dr. Donald L. Cooper, Director of Student Health Service, Oklahoma State University, an enthusiastic wrestling supporter, who kindly gave me material that is of practical benefit to the athlete.

Heartfelt appreciation goes to Dr. and Mrs. Robert L. Smith for their encouragement during several years of creating nutrition materials.

Finally, special love to my children who were like a cheering section, encouraging me via letters, phone, and in person, to "keep on, keeping on." And to my grandchildren, may this book help create a continuing interest in good nutrition, and a realization that nothing is as important as good health. May it be a blessing—much appreciated and cherished throughout their lifetime.

part 1

Feeding the Body

NUTRITION

What is the real meaning of *nutrition?* We probably have heard of it, vaguely, for as long as we can remember. Very likely we have been eating three or more meals a day all of our lives, but have we been inspired to learn what we should be eating?

To say that nutrition is a science dealing with the effects of food on the body *or* nutrition includes the food we eat and how the body uses it, defines the term very simply. Foods vary in their importance to the body; no one food provides all the requirements for growth and good health.

Nutrition has received much publicity in recent years, which has helped to make people at least curious about it. Meal planning, preparation, and eating can be fascinating once we learn *what* our body requires and *how* we can provide the energy needed for all of the activities we undertake.

Questions are numerous from athletes, coaches, and parents

concerning nutrition and physical performance. Too often in past years, the coach made generalizations regarding diet. He would tell his athletes to, "Stick to a sensible diet—no rich foods, no snacking, no fried foods, no starchy foods," and so forth. But who among his athletes knew what a "sensible diet" really was?

Americans—including athletes—of all ages and both sexes are influenced by advertising claims for foods and numerous vitamin-mineral-protein supplements. Health food stores and famous athletes are promoting all kinds of dietary supplements. Many claims are misleading or only partial truths made to sell a product. Acceptance of many unsound, even dangerous eating practices has come about.

Athletes and coaches are concerned about the effects of various dietary regimens on physical performance. Which vitamin should be taken to develop stamina? Should steak be eaten to promote muscle growth? It is encouraging to see the new wave of interest in nutrition.

Needed now are coaches and trainers who have some knowledge of nutrition and the ability to adapt it to an athlete's life and sport. Faddism, ignorance, and just poor eating habits are prevalent in athletics. Athletes might not have paid much attention before, but learning and practicing good nutrition can help them in physical fitness and readiness conditioning as well as promote rapid healing and recovery following injury or illness—all important in attaining the goal of championship performance.

Ignoring nutrition can lead to unnecessary handicaps in striving for athletic excellence. But of far greater importance than athletic championships is a lifetime of good health, promoted through learning and practicing good nutrition.

NUTRIENTS

The term *nutrients* is a convenient word that includes all the components of foods (such as protein, fat, carbohydrates) that the body needs in order to fulfill the three main requirements for life and good health. These requirements are, first, an *energy* supply for body warmth, internal organ function, and body locomotion; second, the ability to *regulate* and *control* body reactions; and third, the power to *build*, *repair*, and *maintain* body tissues.

There are about fifty known nutrients. We can think of *nutrients* as teammates who work together to keep the body healthy and functioning. There is no need to remember the names of fifty nutrients, but it is easy to keep in mind their six classes, each having precise chemical characteristics and each suited to meet specific body needs. The six classes are: *water, carbohydrates, fats, proteins, vitamins,* and *minerals.* Since each nutrient performs specific functions in the body, a lack of just one of them is a disadvantage, just as when a teammate fouls out of the game!

1
Water, Water

Are you surprised that water is a nutrient? It doesn't have the life-giving ability of proteins, the energy sources of carbohydrates and fats, the minute metabolism control qualities of vitamins, or the richness of minerals, but water is essential for life! It ranks next to air (oxygen) in importance.

Water, a simple compound of two atoms of hydrogen with one of oxygen, has unique features. No other chemical compound performs so many distinct and vital functions as water.

FUNCTIONS OF WATER

Water is used as a solvent in the digestive processes, where it aids the chewing and softening of food. It also supplies fluid for the digestive juices and facilitates the movement of the food mass along the digestive tract. After digestion, water, as a constituent of blood, is the means by which nutrients are carried to the cells.

1

Water is essential for flushing away the body's chemical wastes. For example, the use of proteins by the cells leaves a waste called urea. The more protein we eat and the more salt added to our food, the more water we need. The kidneys demand water to flush wastes out of the body. These wastes must be diluted to a certain level in order to be excreted as urine.

Water functions as a building material in the construction of each cell, and the different cells vary in their water content. Water also serves as a lubricant for moving parts such as the joints, for the pumping of the heart, and for the peristalsis of the intestines. As a lubricant it also keeps body cells moist and permits the passage of substances between cells and blood vessels. Water also comprises a large part of the fluid that serves as a cushion for the brain and spinal cord.

Water also plays an indispensable part in the functions of our sense organs. Taste and smell result from the stimulation of chemical compounds in solution. Sound is conducted through the inner ear by a liquid that is chiefly water. The functioning of the semicircular canals, sense organs of balance, is dependent on water. The transparency of the media of the eye to light is maintained by water. Water is important, too, in moistening the surface of the lungs for gas diffusion.

NEED FOR WATER

A regular and generous intake of water is required to perform all of these tasks, which are effortlessly carried on when the water consumed is sufficient. The kidneys and liver are both master filters of the body and especially susceptible to dangerous infections when too little water is taken into the body.

Since the body is mostly water (two-thirds), it needs a fresh supply of liquid each day just to maintain its essential balance and to carry on its functions normally. Between three and four quarts of water (in the form of blood) are constantly being circulated to every cell in the body.

Water is so essential for life that a water loss of 10 percent of total body weight is serious, and a loss of 20 percent may result in a painful death.

SOURCES OF WATER

The body gets water from many sources. The most obvious is the water we drink plus such beverages as tea, coffee, soft drinks, fruit juices, and so forth. But this represents only a small part of the total intake. We get much of our needed water from food. Fruits and vegetables are usually about 85 percent water. Meat contains a quantity of water. Even bread is heavy with about 35 percent moisture.

AMOUNT OF WATER

Adults need about 3 ounces of water for every 100 calories of food consumed. An average athlete, consuming perhaps 4,500 calories daily, needs well over 2 quarts each day. Because of the high water content of food, we do not have to drink all this water, but a quart of water a day is an absolute minimum.

Don't depend on thirst to tell you when water is needed. Form the habit of drinking water regularly, at definite times and in definite amounts. Think water—at least 8 glasses of liquid a day, more according to amount of activity and temperature of the body. Learn to drink water on arising; also drink between meals. Good water is the greatest thirst quencher there is.

With water, unlike food, there is little danger of taking too much. Excess food is stored in the form of fat, but the kidneys simply flush out excess water! You need not worry about drinking too much fluid if your body is in a good state of health because your kidneys will unload the water in a matter of a few hours. A primary concern of athletes should be their water consumption. Remember, water is the body's most urgent need—*it is more important than food!*

TABLE 1-1   PERCENTAGE OF WATER IN SOME COMMONLY USED FOODS*

Food	Percent
Rice, puffed	3.7
Crackers, soda	4.0
Bacon (cooked)	8.1
Raisins (uncooked)	18.0
Bread, white enriched	35.8
Cheese, cheddar	37.0
Steak (broiled)	56.3
Fish (baked)	58.1
Hamburger (cooked)	60.0
Broiler chicken	71.0
Ice cream (12 percent)	63.2
Eggs (hard cooked)	73.7
Potatoes, white (baked)	75.1
Bananas	75.7
Gelatin dessert	84.2
Most fruits (fresh)	86.0
Most vegetables (fresh)	87.0
Milk, skim	90.5
Watermelon	92.6
Lettuce, iceberg	95.5

*Figures from Agriculture Handbook No. 8, United States Department of Agriculture, Rev. Oct. 1975.

2

Carbohydrates— Food for Fuel

Carbohydrates are the most efficient and usually the least expensive source of food energy. Carbohydrates are almost entirely the product of plants. Photosynthesis is the process by which sunlight helps plants make carbohydrates from carbon dioxide and water.

No one knows exactly how photosynthesis works, for it is extremely complicated. But two things are known to happen. First, light is used by the chlorophyll in the plant to split water taken from the soil into hydrogen and oxygen. Second, the hydrogen, raised to a high level of energy by sunlight, combines with carbon dioxide taken from the air to form starches and sugars, the bases of all carbohydrates. If scientists could learn to do what a plant does with carbon dioxide, light, and water, they could make simple carbohydrates.

A chemical analysis of carbohydrates reveals that the elements of hydrogen and oxygen are present (with the carbon) in the same two-to-one proportion as in water (H_2O);

5

thus, a carbohydrate is a hydrate of carbon. The simplest carbohydrate, sugar, has the formula $C_6H_{12}O_6$.

SUGARS

Simple sugars form the basis for all carbohydrates, and all of these compounds that occur commonly in food are either six-carbon sugar ($C_6H_{12}O_6$) or multiples of six-carbon sugar groups.

Carbohydrates are subdivided into three groups according to the complexity and size of their molecules. The three classes are known as simple sugars, or *monosaccharides* (one sugar group per molecule), *disaccharides* (two sugar groups per molecule) and *polysaccharides* (many sugar groups per molecule).

The most important carbohydrates in the diet and the groups to which they belong are as follows: *glucose, fructose,* and *galactose* are monosaccharides (simple sugars); *sucrose, maltose,* and *lactose are disaccharides (double sugars); starch, dextrins, glycogen,* and *cellulose* are polysaccharides (many sugars).

Carbohydrates that are disaccharides and polysaccharides must be broken down by digestion into the simple sugar groups such as glucose before they can be absorbed and used by the body. All food carbohydrates are formed in the plant kingdom except two, which are from the animal kingdom: lactose in milk and glycogen in liver.

Monosaccharides (simple sugars)

GLUCOSE is a simple sugar, but very little, as such, occurs in our daily diet. The body makes all it needs from starch and from proteins.

FRUCTOSE is a simple sugar that occurs chiefly in fruit and plant juices. It is about three times as sweet as glucose and can replace ordinary sugar in all foods.

GALACTOSE is a simple sugar derived from lactose.

Disaccharides (double sugars)

SUCROSE is a common table sugar, a disaccharide made of glucose and fructose. It is found chiefly in the juice of sugar cane or sugar beets. The sugars from these two sources are identical chemically. Refined sugar is an unusual food in that it is pure carbohydrate without vitamins, minerals, protein, or fat; it is a source of calories only, or "empty" calories. Almost all other foods contain some combination of essential nutrients.

MALTOSE is an intermediate product formed in the process of breaking down starch to glucose. When you see "maltose" on a label, you know you are getting carbohydrates. We use maltoses to make flavoring and in making beers and whiskies. The main use of barley today is to make malt for these purposes.

LACTOSE is a milk sugar. Lactose occurs in the milk of most mammals and serves as the source of energy for the young. On digestion, it is broken down into glucose and galactose.

Polysaccharides (many sugars)

STARCH is the carbohydrate found in seeds, tubers, and roots, where it serves as an energy store for future use by the plant.

DEXTRINS are partly broken down starches. They are intermediate products formed in the process of breaking down starch to glucose. Dextrins are more soluble than starch, and their molecules average about one-fifth the size of those of starch.

GLYCOGEN is sometimes called "animal starch" because it is the polysaccharide stored in animal tissues instead of starch. Glycogen is the storage form of carbohydrates in man and is found in muscle tissue and the liver.

CELLULOSE is a large, complex carbohydrate that makes up the structural or fibrous part of plants, including leaves, stems, roots, seeds, and fruit coverings. Leafy vegetables such as lettuce and cabbage and stem vegetables such as celery are high in cellulose.

Other Sweeteners

BROWN SUGAR is a sucrose. It is slightly more nutritious than white sugar because it acquires from the molasses that colors it potassium and minute amounts of minerals such as calcium and iron. Whether it is deep brown or merely tan depends on the amount of molasses in the sugar.

HONEY is a sweetener with no special health value other than minute amounts of vitamins and minerals. Fructose and glucose occur in honey in about fifty-fifty proportions. It has no special energy-producing value beyond that of other sugar products. And one kind of honey does not have more food value than another kind; they all are just sweeteners!

MOLASSES is a source of potassium, lesser amounts of calcium and iron, and minute amounts of other minerals; but it, too, is just a sweetener!

CORN SYRUP is a sugar that is included in many of our foods only to make them taste better! Read the food labels to determine how many foods have corn syrup in them.

MAPLE SUGAR is the sugar obtained from the sap of the sugar maple tree. It consists of fructose and glucose and has no special health value either.

HEALTHFUL SOURCES OF CARBOHYDRATES

FRUITS: All kinds, both fresh and dried, including dates, figs, raisins, prunes, apricots, apples, peaches, pineapple, grapefruit, oranges, bananas, and melons of all kinds.

VEGETABLES: All kinds, including tubers (such as potatoes) and roots (such as carrots). All types of lettuce, cabbages, etc.

LEGUMES: All kinds of beans and peas (also high in protein and therefore good meat substitutes).

CEREAL GRAINS: All varieties such as wheat, corn, rye, buck-
wheat, millet, rice, etc., (whole, cracked, or ground).

SEEDS AND NUTS: All kinds, including sunflower, pumpkin,
almonds, cashews, walnuts, filberts, etc.

CARBOHYDRATE FOOD PRODUCTS: Bread, waffles, pancakes,
pies, spaghetti, macaroni, etc. Many of these foods are
relatively inexpensive, but there is a popular notion that
they are of low nutritional value. Not true—they can be
most nutritious.

There need be no health hazard in subsisting chiefly on
carbohydrate foods provided those foods are not lacking in
proteins, minerals, and vitamins or provided that the diet
includes some other rich sources of these nutrients.

Soft drinks, cakes, cookies, doughnuts, candies, syrups, jams,
jellies, and many other sweet "man-made" products have a
high sugar content. But many of these foods contribute
calories without providing much in the way of nutrients.
These calorie-laden carbohydrates cannot take the place of
whole grain cereals, legumes, fruits, and vegetables.

Just remember, there is a limit to the amount of carbohydrates our bodies can use as energy or can store as energy.
The surplus is *stored as fat!* Excess calories from any source—
protein, fat, or carbohydrate—lead to overweight!

IMPORTANCE OF CARBOHYDRATES

There are no definite requirements for carbohydrates as there
are for some nutrients such as protein, nor can it be said that
any special level of carbohydrate intake is most conducive to
health. But the following indicates the importance of carbohydrates to body needs.

Carbohydrates are more quickly mobilized as energy fuel
than are proteins and fats.

In humans, fat cannot be oxidized properly without
carbohydrates.

Carbohydrates assist proteins in making "nonessential"

amino acids. "Nonessential" means that the body can make them; see Chapter 4.

Carbohydrates are found in combination with some proteins and often provide necessary minerals and vitamins. (Milk is a good example.)

Carbohydrates are especially important to cardiac muscle, where a constant supply of fuel is vital.

Glucose, the simplest and most common sugar, is the source of fuel for the brain and nervous system and is a necessary food if they are to function properly.

Fructose is completely and rapidly absorbed into the bloodstream and then quickly converted into glycogen for storage if it is not needed immediately for energy.

Glycogen is the form in which energy is stored in the liver.

Lactose and some other carbohydrates provide sustenance for bacteria in the intestine, where they produce small amounts of some of the B-complex vitamins.

Lactose serves in the utilization of calcium and other minerals. The enzyme lactase must be present to digest lactose. Some people are deficient or lacking in this enzyme after early childhood and find it difficult or are unable to digest milk or milk products containing lactose.

Most of the fibrous material of plant foods, cellulose, is only softened by cooking processes and cannot be digested by our bodies. Cellulose is, therefore, not an energy source as are all other carbohydrates, but the material is needed to give bulk to food residues in the intestines. Cellulose supplies the roughage needed for proper elimination of solid wastes from the body.

STARCH

Sugars are very soluble in water; they are the form in which plants transport carbohydrates from one part of the plant to another via the sap or tuck it away for temporary storage in the juices of fruits. If you have tasted fresh corn and peas, you will remember how sweet they are; as vegetables mature, the sugar is converted to starch.

Starchy foods are not very flavorful if eaten raw. Cooking swells starch granules, breaks them open, makes them taste better, and allows them to be digested more easily. Raw potatoes, for example, are a favorite of very few, but a baked potato can be a gourmet delight.

Before starch can be used as a source of energy, either in the plant or in the body, it first must be broken down into the simple sugar groups of which it is composed, each starch molecule yielding many molecules of glucose. Dextrins and maltose are intermediate products formed in the process of breaking starch back down to the simple sugar, glucose.

WHOLE GRAIN REFINEMENT

Cereals contain principally starch, but important vitamins and minerals are present in the outer layer and the germ of the grain or kernel.

When grains are milled (refined), the outer layer (bran) and the embryo (germ) of the grain seed are removed. The protein and starch remain. The milled, or refined, product is what we know as "flour." Less refined grains such as whole wheat flours contain more nutrients than highly refined white flour.

Enrichment of white bread and flour restores three of the B vitamins that are lost in processing and also adds iron, but the minute amounts of many vitamins and minerals from the bran layer and the germ part of the kernels are not restored. Therefore, it is a good idea to eat some whole grain foods often rather than depend entirely on enriched products for vitamins and minerals.

SUMMARY

Carbohydrates are the products of plants. With the help of sunlight, plants are able to take carbon from the carbon dioxide in the air, and combine it with water from the soil to make a nutrient called carbohydrate. The elements of hydrogen and oxygen are always present (with carbon) in the same two-to-one proportion as in water.

TABLE 2-1   GOOD CARBOHYDRATE FOOD SOURCES*

Food Sources	Percent Carbohydrate
FRUITS (dried)	
Apricots, apples, bananas, raisins	80 to 85
CEREALS (dry)	80 to 85
BREADS and ROLLS (enriched)	50
PASTA (cooked)	
Macaroni, spaghetti, noodles, also rice (all enriched)	25 to 30
POTATOES	
Sweet, white, also sweet winter squash	15 to 30
LEGUMES	20 to 25
FRUITS (fresh)	15 to 23
CEREALS (cooked)	10
VEGETABLES (raw or cooked)	5 to 10
LIVER	5.3
MILK (skim)	5.1

* Figures from Agriculture Handbook No. 8, United States Department of Agriculture, approved for reprinting October 1975.

Simple sugars form the basis of all carbohydrates, and all the sugars that occur commonly in food are either six-carbon sugar or multiples of six-carbon sugar. Carbohydrates are divided into three groups: simple sugars, or monosaccharides (one sugar group per molecule), disaccharides (two sugar groups per molecule), and polysaccharides (many sugar groups per molecule).

Monosaccharides include glucose, fructose, and galactose; disaccharides include sucrose, maltose, and lactose; and polysaccharides include starch, dextrin, glycogen, and cellulose. Carbohydrates that are disaccharides and polysaccharides must be broken down by digestion into simple sugars such as glucose before they can be absorbed and used by the body.

Carbohydrates are found in great variety and include the most nutritious of foods: fruits of all kinds, vegetables (including leafy greens as well as potatoes), legumes, cereal grains of all varieties, seeds, and a wonderful array of nuts. Carbohydrates also include manmade sweets such as candies, cookies, cakes, and soft drinks, which are *high in calories*, but *low in nutrients*. These calories are known as "empty calories."

Athletes should know that carbohydrates also provide the most efficient energy fuel in the body. They are needed in the metabolism of fat and for energy, to assist proteins in the formation of amino acids, to furnish necessary fuel for the brain and nervous system, to serve as a short-time energy reserve, and to assist in vitamin and mineral functions of the body. We are increasingly more aware, and should be, of the importance of carbohydrates in our diet. They are among the most nutritious of foods.

3
Fats—Not Fancy

Mention the word "fat" to people and usually they feel that it is something to avoid if at all possible. Yet fat is an important food. Without fat both plants and animals would die. Our body requires a little fat each day, and the quality of that fat is critical to good health; but most of us have no need to consume one-quarter pound (114 grams) of fat daily, in one form or another, as we now do.

Fats are made by both plants and animals: they serve as a compact way to store fuel. Plants store energy in the form of starch and fat in seeds, seed germs, nuts, and even the fruit itself; animals store fat in their body tissues.

Vegetable oils are important fats. These oils include olive, corn germ, cotton seed, soybean, peanut, coconut, etc. Fats of animal origin are butter, lard, fatty meat and fish, egg yolk, cream, and full-milk cheese.

Fish (of all varieties) store fat (instead of glycogen as humans do) in their liver. That is the source of the fish-liver oils that are widely used for their valuable content of fat-soluble vitamins.

As we think about food for our bodies, we need to be aware of how closely fats, carbohydrates, and proteins work together and depend on each other within each cell and in all the functions that the body performs. The utilization of food in the body is a true miracle. We need a knowledge of food, and we need to eat good food in order to cooperate with our body in this life-preserving effort.

VISIBLE-INVISIBLE FATS

Generally, fat from animals tends to be hard; fat from vegetable sources is likely to be in liquid form, known as oils.

We recognize foods such as butter, lard, salad oil, etc., both liquid and hard, as *visible* fat. We can rather easily determine how much of them we include in our daily eating, but most of us are not aware of the quantity of *invisible* fat we ingest. Even though we think we trim all the visible fat from meat, a choice cut of beef steak is "marbled" with fat. The fat gives it a good flavor as well as juiciness. Instead of pure protein, as an athlete might think he is getting, a steak is often high in fat content—hard animal fat, at that.

Invisible fat also is present in milk. The fact that fat is insoluble in and lighter than water is readily apparent when we observe that fat in whole milk separates from the heavier watery portion and rises to the top if left standing. The older generation might remember the "cream line" on milk. We could pour off the cream if we didn't want to drink it. Most fresh milk now sold is homogenized, that is, put through a process that breaks up the fat into such fine particles that it remains evenly distributed in the fluid. Fat that is in small droplets in a fluid, as in milk, is more quickly digested because the tiny droplets can be surrounded and attacked by digestive juices.

Other not-so-visible fats include the fat that the cook adds to our food "to make it taste good," such as butter in a cooked vegetable, and we must remember that there is fat—many times, a lot of it—in the commercially processed "goodies" we consume.

Fruits and vegetables are almost free of fat, except for the rich stores of fat "hidden" in avocados and olives. Nuts of all kinds are a vital treasure chest of fat.

FATTY ACIDS OF FATS

Fats contain large amounts of carbon and hydrogen and smaller amounts of oxygen, in combination with glycerin and certain acids. Therefore, fats sometimes are called glycerides of fatty acids. The most important of the fatty acids are palmitic, stearic, and oleic acids. There are comparatively large amounts of palmitic and stearic acids in hard fats while liquid fats, such as olive and cotton seed oils, contain more oleic acids. Oleic acid is found in relatively large amounts in oils—along with variable amounts of polyunsaturated fatty acids.

SATURATED AND UNSATURATED FATS

Fats are classified according to the saturation or unsaturation of the fatty acids. Saturation is determined by how many places exist on the fatty acid molecule for additional atoms of hydrogen. A fatty acid that has no room for hydrogen is called *saturated*. Most animal fats are saturated and usually are solid at room temperature. Bacon fat and other meat fats, butter, lard, and even cream are examples of saturated fats.

Monounsaturates

A fatty acid that can take two more hydrogen atoms is *monounsaturated*. A chemical treatment of unsaturated fatty acids allows the compound to incorporate more hydrogen atoms; by this process, oils can be converted to a semisolid or solid state.

Hydrogenation is the modern food technology process whereby vegetable oils are converted into a semisolid state for use as cooking fats (lard substitutes) and margarines of varying degrees of softness. Two vegetable oils predominate in momonounsaturates: peanut oil and olive oil.

Polyunsaturates

A fatty acid that has room for four or more additional hydrogen atoms is *polyunsaturated*. The polyunsaturated fats have great nutritional value. *Linoleic, linolenic,* and *arachidonic acids* all are polyunsaturated. Vegetable oils high in polyunsaturates include safflower, sunflower, corn, soybean, peanut, and cotton seed. The labels on products made from these oils will state: "High in polyunsaturates" or "High in polyunsaturated fatty acids."

Linoleic Acid

Linoleic acid is of particular nutritional importance because the body cannot manufacture it; thus, it is an "essential" fatty acid because it must be supplied in the food we eat. Linoleic acid is needed for growth, a healthy skin, and general well being. The need for linoleic acid is similar to the need for vitamins, but it is not a vitamin.

The amount of linoleic acid in most fats of animal origin is only low to moderate. Include pork, beef, and lamb—with their fat—in order to obtain some linoleic acid from an animal source. Oil from plants such as corn, cotton seed, soybean, wheat germ, and safflower are especially rich in linoleic acid. Other good sources are peanut oil, margarine, and vegetable shortenings. Linoleic acid is not present in olive or coconut oil.

Only a small amount of linoleic acid is required to meet the daily need. One can figure the daily need at about six grams per day or one to two percent of the total calories consumed. Very simply, if a person has a minimum of one to two tablespoons of polyunsaturated fat, a good vegetable oil preferred, the need for linoleic acid should be met.

TABLE 3-1 FOOD SOURCES AND PERCENTAGES OF LINOLEIC ACID

Foods	Percent
Safflower oil	72
Corn oil	53
Soybean oil	52
Cottonseed oil	50
Peanutbutter	42 to 49
Sesame oil	42
English walnuts	40
Mayonnaise (corn, cottonseed, soy oil, and veg.)	40
Sunflower seeds	30
Peanut oil	29
Salad dressing (corn, cottonseed, soy oil)	25
Peanuts, shelled	14
Soybean flour (full fat)	11

*Figures from Agriculture Handbook No. 8, United States Department of Agriculture, approved for reprinting October, 1975.

LIPIDS OTHER THAN TRUE FATS

Some substances have physical properties similar to fats, i.e., they are oily and greasy, and are called *lipids*. A lipid that has received much attention is *lecithin*. It is formed by the union of one molecule of glycerol, two molecules of fatty acid, and one molecule each of phosphoric acid and choline, a nitrogenous base. Lecithin, a phospholipid, is prominent in egg yolks and found also in soybeans. Choline that is present in lecithin is known to be used in metabolizing fats; it is a component of one of the most important chemicals helping the nervous system to function, and it participates in the body's synthesis of proteins.

Since lecithin is an emulsifier, it has received wide publicity in health magazines and health food stores as an antidote to high blood cholesterol and heart disease. Lecithin cannot dissolve the plaques in blood vessels—as health food "experts" may claim. Problems associated with high blood cholesterol and heart attacks cannot be solved by taking lecithin in powder or pill form.

Role of Lipids

The various lipids play extremely important roles in many enzyme reactions, in cell membrane structure, in the synthesis and regulation of certain hormones, in the maintenance of the proper structure of blood vessels, and in energy metabolism digestion, tissue structure, nerve impulse transmission, and memory storage, to name several.

Cholesterol

Another group of lipids, in addition to the phospholipids, consists of the sterols, which are complex solid alcohols. *Cholesterol* is the most prominent member of this group. Phospholipids, including lecithin, and sterols, including cholesterol, are widely distributed in small amounts in foods. Cholesterol is a *normal* constituent of blood plasma and body tissues in man. It is a fatty substance found in all animal fats and oils, but cholesterol is most concentrated in egg yolk and liver. It is not found in plants; therefore, vegetable oils have no cholesterol.

Cholesterol is a complex fat that animal cells (including those of man) can synthesize from building blocks provided by the metabolism of carbohydrates and fats. After six months of age, the body can synthesize all the cholesterol it needs; therefore, the consumption of foods containing cholesterol is not necessary. Approximately two grams are synthesized each day within the body of a normal adult.

Valuable Role of Cholesterol

Cholesterol is essential to the body. It plays a vital role in healthy, everyday life, and without it we would be in sorry shape! These are some of the roles cholesterol plays:

Cholesterol is a necessary part of the structure of cell membranes.

Cholesterol is an important factor in the production of sex and adrenal hormones for the healthy functioning of the reproductive system. (Cholesterol serves as a precursor in their synthesis.)

Cholesterol covers the long nerve cells and acts as an aid to the conduction of nerve impulses throughout the body. Any deficiency in cholesterol within the body can precipitate a wide variety of malfunctions within the nervous system.

Cholesterol is an important link in the chain of events that eventually produces vitamin D in our body. (This vitamin often is referred to as the "sunshine" vitamin.) The cholesterol contained within the skin undergoes a conversion when the ultraviolet light in sunlight penetrates the skin.

Cholesterol is a substance that is *normal* in the body and *useful* to the body.

Waxes

Waxes are included among the lipids and normally are present in very small amounts in many foods, usually of vegetable origin. Wax is a hard, brittle, fatty substance obtained from animal, vegetable, and mineral sources. Nature provides most plants, flowers, and fruits with a shield of wax. We might not see the natural wax coating, but sometimes we can feel a

slight waxiness on fruits and vegetables; most o/ [...]
are not even aware of it. The wax layer seals in [...]
moisture and helps prevent damage from the sun's hot ray[...]
young plants and fruit. Wax is not easily affected by exposure
to the air, and rain does not destroy its protective value.

Most honey is marketed in the "strained" state in jars, but
bees deposit their honey in a "comb." The comb is an
example of edible wax in our diet when we eat honey in this
form. There is no particular value or harm for a healthy
person to ingest this kind of vegetable wax.

FUNCTIONS OF FAT—HOW FAT HELPS US

1. Fat is a source of the "essential" fatty acids linoleic.
2. Fat serves as a carrier of fat-soluble vitamins A, D, E, and K.
3. Fat serves as a concentrated source of energy.
4. Fat helps make food more appetizing.
5. Fat has satiety value—feeling of fullness after eating.
6. Fat tissue serves to insulate and to cushion organs of the body.

Fat As a Source of "Essential" Fatty Acid—Linoleic

The most important use of fat in the diet is as a source of the
"essential" fatty acid, linoleic. Carbohydrates, or even proteins, can substitute for fats in other ways but not in providing
linoleic.

There is a class of vital hormone-like compounds made in
various tissues of the body from some derivatives of linoleic
acid that are important in the regulation of gastric secretion,
in pancreatic functions, in the release of pituitary hormones,
and in smooth muscle metabolism. Because of this, we should
realize that fats no longer can be considered simply a source
of energy for body heat and work—they are far more important.

Animal fats are more limited in the "essential" fatty acid

than are vegetable fats. Among animal fats, beef and pork are a little higher in their "essential" fatty acid content than some other foods, but we must eat the lean and the fat on the meat to get the fatty acid.

Vegetable oils are the best sources; these are contained in a number of commonly prepared foods such as mayonnaise made from the oil of corn, safflower, soybean, etc., or salad dressing made from vegetable oil. Some baked products also contain vegetable oils.

In general, the "essential" fatty acid tends to appear with other polyunsaturated fatty acids.

How Much Fatty Acid Do We Need?

There is no set allowance for the "essential" fatty acid, but the Food and Nutrition Board suggests that a linoleic acid intake equivalent to nearly two percent of the total calories in the diet should be sufficient for adults. A person who requires 2,500 calories a day would need only about 50 calories worth of linoleic acid. An average amount needed is equivalent to 1 to 2 tablespoons of polyunsaturated oils. A typical American diet includes at least that much linoleic acid. Most of us need not be concerned that we're not consuming enough, but if one is on a self-prescribed fat-free or very low-fat diet, one should be aware of the daily need for a small amount of linoleic acid. It is sensible to include fat in one's diet and not to think of a small amount of fat as villainous.

Carriers of Important Vitamins

Fat is important in the absorption and transportation of fat-soluble vitamins A, D, E, and K. These four vitamins are soluble in fat and fat solvents. Fat-soluble vitamins are absorbed from the intestine along with fats and lipids in foods, so anything that interferes with fat absorption results in a lowered utilization of this class of vitamin. The presence of fat favors their absorption.

Fat as a Source of Energy

Fat formerly was considered *only* a source of heat and energy. Fat is useful when it is desirable to have a higher intake of food energy without adding unduly to the bulk of the diet. Fat furnishes more than twice as much fuel and energy for the body as the same amount of carbohydrate because fat contains more carbon and hydrogen. Fat is a concentrated source of calories (energy)—9 calories per gram as opposed to 4 per gram from protein or carbohydrate. A pure fat has a fuel value of 4,040 calories per pound while sugar, a typical carbohydrate, has a fuel value of only 1,820 calories per pound.

Most fats are digested at about the same rate whether they are in the form of butter, margarine, salad dressing, shortening, or in the natural content of food. The normal athlete can successfully digest food fried in fat; moderate amounts of fried foods are not taboo for the athlete.

A diet very low in fat often supplies less energy than the body needs, thereby resulting in weight loss. If one overeats fats, the diet very likely will provide food energy in excess of body needs, and undesirable weight gain will result.

Excess energy value of the diet, whether in the form of fat, carbohydrate, or protein, is converted into body fat to be stored in fatty tissues in various parts of the body. All fat not used for fuel energy or growth is stored in the tissues as body fat. Some deposition of fat, usually under the skin or around the abdominal organs, serves a useful purpose as a reserve store of fuel to be drawn on in time of need. Fat is the primary source of reserve fuel. It is a concentrated energy source appropriate for long-term storage of energy, but the conversion process involved in energy utilization is more complicated than that for carbohydrates. Consequently, energy from fat is not as readily available.

Appetizing and Satiety Value

Fats incorporated and naturally present in foods make them

more palatable by enhancing flavor and texture. Salad oils, dressing, butter, and spreads all help to make food more palatable and satisfying. When one is on a reducing diet, small amounts of fat are a help in preventing hunger.

The satiety value of fats depends on their slow digestion and thus the emptying time of the stomach. Since fats are absorbed in the body over a period of four to six hours—far more slowly than proteins or carbohydrates—they help to reduce hunger between meals. But when too much fat is taken, the meal might remain in the stomach too long and cause discomfort.

Fat Deposits as Protection and Insulation

Any excess energy in the body, whether derived from carbohydrate, fat, proteins or alcohol, is stored as fat within adipose cells.

Fat cushions vital organs of the body, supporting some organs and offering protection against jars and stresses. Since fat is a poor conductor of heat, moderate deposits of fatty tissue also serve to insulate and to prevent undue loss of heat from the body surface. This enables the body to maintain a nearly constant temperature.

It is important, however, to maintain only as much fat as is needed for protection and insulation.

HOW FAT HURTS US

Fat deposits in the human body can be either advantageous or disadvantageous, depending on whether they are moderate or excessive. An overfed person stores fat that he may never need to burn as body fuel; such excessive fat deposits result in undesirable weight gains and place undue strain on the heart and other vital organs. Insurance company figures show that overweight persons have a much lower life expectancy than those who maintain normal weight for their height and age.

PLACE OF FAT-RICH FOODS IN THE DIET

The amount of fat in the diet may be varied, as is the case for carbohydrate intake, according to personal tastes, money available for food, and availability of fat-rich foods.

In the United States as much as 40 to 45 percent of the energy content of the diet might come from fat-rich foods. Since we are a people guilty of over-consumption of food and, as a result, inclined to overweight and heart attacks, we are urged to lower our fat intake. Eating some saturated fats is permissible, but choosing a variety of fats to provide sufficient unsaturated fatty acids is encouraged.

Many nutritionists suggest that fats should not account for more than about one-third of the calories we take in and perhaps only one-fourth. That gives us an eating pattern of about 15 percent protein, 52 to 60 percent carbohydrate, and 25 to 33 percent fat. Of the 25 to 33 percent fat, less than 10 percent of the total calories should come from saturated fatty acids and at least 10 percent from polyunsaturated fatty acids. This would provide a diet conducive to better health in the U.S. population.

DIETS TOO LOW IN FAT

Perhaps one also should be warned that diets too low in fat are not desirable either. When the diet is very low in fats or practically fat-free because of unavailability of fatty foods or because of restriction for weight reduction or other therapeutic purposes, the average person does not increase his consumption of carbohydrates and proteins sufficiently to furnish equivalent energy; thus, he will lose weight and may have less vigor. "Essential" fatty acids and most fat-soluble vitamins gain entrance to the body through fat intake, so a low-fat diet could result in less than adequate amounts of these important nutrients. Reducing diets that are low in fat probably need to be supplemented with foods containing vitamin A or, if on an extended diet, supplemented with vitamin A in capsule form to meet the 5,000 International Unit (IU) daily requirement.

FAT REQUIREMENT

As far as nutrition is concerned, saturated fats are not needed in the diet. Polyunsaturates supply one "essential" dietary fatty acid, and both poly- and monounsaturates can transport fat-soluble vitamins. Except for these needs, there is no specific requirement for fat as a nutrient in the diet.

FAT FOR THE ATHLETE

There appears to be no sound rationale for the inclusion of increased amounts of fat in the diet of an athlete. Fat is not a readily available source of energy, although it will provide some energy for endurance events. Nevertheless, the athlete, like all individuals, must have an adequate daily fat intake. Most food fats, of either animal or vegetable origin, are readily digested by healthy persons.

FOOD LABELING

From a nutritional point of view, it is important to know the kind and fatty acid composition of the fat one is consuming. It is hoped that labeling of manufactured food products is providing helpful information, but information concerning fats is especially important to many people. Be a label reader—know what fats are in your foods!

SUMMARY

Fats are available from both plant and animal sources. They serve as compact fuel storage. Fruits and vegetables are almost free of fat. Fats are classified as saturated or unsaturated. Animal fats usually are saturated and solid at room temperature. Fats that are soft or liquid in form are unsaturated; they are usually vegetable fats or oils.

Linoleic acid is an important fatty acid that cannot be manufactured in the body. It must be supplied in the food we eat; therefore, it is an "essential" fatty acid. Corn, cottonseed, soybean, wheat germ, and safflower oils are especially rich in linoleic acid. The body needs about one to two tablespoons of polyunsaturated oil each day.

Cholesterol is a substance that is normal and useful to the body. Avoid consuming unnecessary amounts of it because the body manufactures it.

For the sake of good health, limit the amount of fat deposited in your body.

4

Proteins—Without Peer

Proteins have been described as the most complex chemical compounds known. They form larger and more complex molecules than those of either fats or carbohydrates. All three nutrients—carbohydrates, fats, and proteins—contain carbon, hydrogen, and oxygen, but in addition proteins contain nitrogen, an element indispensable for life and growth.

By a process called photosynthesis, plants can build their own protein. They are able to take nitrogen from the soil, hydrogen and oxygen from water absorbed directly by the roots, and carbon from the air to make nitrogen-containing substances.

Plants can use nitrates from the soil, and some bacteria can take nitrogen from the air, but man and other animals cannot utilize these simple sources of nitrogen for making protein; they must get their protein ready-made. This means that animals are dependent upon plants and other animals for their source of nitrogen, which is in the protein they eat.

Animals get protein (and thus nitrogen) by eating plants (grasses and legumes) and other animal tissue. Man also obtains protein directly from plants by eating legumes (such as dried peas and beans, soybeans, and peanuts), cereals and nuts, animal products (milk, eggs, cheese), and body tissues of animals (meat of all kinds). Each animal, including man, takes protein, in whatever form it is offered, and breaks it down by digestion into amino acids.

AMINO ACIDS

Amino acid is the name given to any of a group of nitrogenous organic compounds that make up an essential part of all the proteins in the tissues of living things. Amino acids are called the "building blocks" of proteins. They all contain carbon, hydrogen, oxygen, and nitrogen, and most contain sulfur and small amounts of other minerals.

Amino acids contain at least one molecule of an amino radical and one molecule called an organic acid. The amino radical consists of two hydrogen atoms attached to a nitrogen atom (NH_2); the organic acid is made of one carbon atom, two oxygen atoms, and one hydrogen atom (COOH).

There are twenty different amino acids available as building blocks for proteins. These twenty amino acids are divided into two groups, "essential" and "nonessential." One of these groups contains eight chemical structures that the human body cannot duplicate but that adults absolutely must have to live. This group is known as the "essential" amino acids, which means that it is essential that they be included directly in the diet. For young children, two additional amino acids, histidine and arginine, are regarded as dietary essentials. The young body can make them, but there is a problem of quantity. During certain phases of life, such as the years of growth, the limited amounts the body can make may not be enough. However, these two aminos are included in the list of "nonessential" amino acids listed below in alphabetical order.

"Essential" Amino Acids	*"Nonessential"* Amino Acids
Isoleucine	Alanine
Leucine	Arginine*
Lysine	Aspartic acid
Methionine	Histidine*
Phenylalanine	Cysteine
Threonine	Cystine
Tryptophan	Glutamic acid
Valine	Glycine
	Hydroxyproline
	Proline
	Serine
	Tyrosine

*"Essential" for young children.

The remaining ten amino acids, plus arginine and histidine, make up the second group and are considered "nonessential". This does not mean we can do without them. It means that the body can build them from the simple elements of which they consist: hydrogen and oxygen (in sugars, starches, and fats) and nitrogen and sulfur (in protein foods). When protein foods are taken into the body, they are digested, or broken up into simple amino acids. The body then reassembles the amino acids into new combinations (molecules). The amino acids are joined together in an intricate pattern characteristic of each individual protein. The *kinds* of amino acids may vary, and the relative *quantities* of each may vary. Thus, the number of individual proteins that it is possible to construct is almost infinite; it is beyond the human mind to comprehend the possibilities. The more knowledge we gain of proteins, the more we are in awe of their complexity and importance.

COMPLETE PROTEINS

Proteins differ greatly in food value, depending upon their

amino acid composition. Proteins that contain all eight of the "essential" amino acids in sufficient amounts are capable of supporting growth and maintaining the tissues of the body. These are called high quality proteins, or *complete* proteins. In general, proteins that come from animal sources are complete proteins. These sources include meat, especially lean meat and liver, fish, poultry, milk, eggs, and cheese. Soybeans and nuts also rank high in both the quality and quantity of their protein content.

INCOMPLETE PROTEINS

Proteins that do not contain all eight "essential" amino acids are called *incomplete proteins*. The proteins of vegetables such as legumes (dried beans and peas) and grains (corn, wheat, rice, oats, etc.) usually are incomplete. These proteins cannot be depended upon individually to support growth and maintain health; they must be supplemented.

One can combine a complete protein such as milk, cheese, or eggs with an incomplete protein such as macaroni, cereal, or bread and enjoy the benefits of a complete protein. When macaroni and cheese, bread and milk, or cereal and milk are eaten *together*, the protein is just as useful to the body (i.e., it can be utilized as completely) as the protein in meat! (A real protein money-saver.)

A varied diet limited to vegetables, grains, and fruits can adequately meet human needs for protein. However, the needs will be met somewhat less efficiently when there is no animal protein in the diet, and consequently larger amounts of vegetable protein will be needed. When just a small amount of animal protein is added to a predominately vegetable diet, the additional amino acid contribution, even though modest, enhances the protein efficiency of the vegetable proteins in the diet. A large number of people take advantage of this fact by adding egg, cheese, or other dairy products to an otherwise strictly vegetarian diet, thus satisfying their protein needs with a so-called "lacto-ovo-vegetarian diet."

Incomplete proteins

Breads made of cracked and whole grains
Soybeans, split peas, navy beans, kidney beans, etc.
Peanuts and peanut butter
Pumpkin, squash, sunflower, sesame and other seeds
Fruits in combination with grains, dairy products, nuts and seeds
Vegetables, including potatoes, both sweet and white
Cashews, almonds, filberts, walnuts, Brazil nuts, etc.
Variety of cereal grains for dry and cooked cereal
Enriched flour for making pasta (noodles, macaroni, spaghetti, etc.,)
Wheat germ, soya milk, and other enrichment of protein.

Complete Proteins

Poultry
Fish
Meat (including organ meats)
Cheese (including both hard and soft)
Eggs
Milk
add to Incomplete Proteins to make a COMPLETE PROTEIN

THE PRINCIPAL FUNCTIONS OF PROTEIN

Proteins are present in all living tissues—plant and animal. In the human body proteins make up between one-half and three-fourths of all solid matter and about one-fifth of total body weight. They are the major organic materials as well as the most important constituents of blood. They are a vital part of the nucleus and protoplasm of every cell as well as the means by which cells are interrelated to one another. The variations of protein in a cell determine its nature, properties, and function. The principal uses of proteins in the body include the following seven functions.

1. To Build New Body Tissues

Proteins are essential for building new tissue. Extra proteins are especially needed during the growing period. An athlete in training may require extra protein for building muscle tissue because muscles strengthen and enlarge as a result of exercise. But remember, muscles do not grow without exercise no matter how much protein one consumes.

Protein provides nourishment for the growth of skin, hair, and nails, as well as for the development and growth of connective tissues, cartilage, tendons, and bones. Increased quantities of protein are needed following bone fractures and surgical operations. Extra protein also is needed following severe hemorrhages.

2. To Maintain Body Tissues

A car is sent to a garage for repairs when a part is worn out, but the human machine must be repaired while it is running since it is never shut down throughout life. All tissues need constant repairing and replacing. The lining of the intestinal tract is renewed about every day and a half; much of this cellular protein is absorbed, but some cells are lost in fecal matter. Blood cells have a limited life span of 120 days, and if replacement protein is not adequate for formation of new cells, anemia develops. Therefore, amino acids and nitrogen are required continuously to replace losses even after body growth has ceased. There are some tissues that never stop growing even when one is old; skin, hair, and nails are obvious examples.

3. To Regulate Body Functions

Proteins exert an important influence on the exchange of water between tissue cells and surrounding body fluids and upon the water balance of the body as a whole. After a prolonged reduced intake of proteins, there is a low protein content in the blood serum. Under such conditions, extra water is retained in the tissues, which become puffy and swollen, making supply of nutrients to the cells and removal of cellular waste products less efficient. This condition is known as low-protein, or nutritional, edema.

A second regulatory function of proteins is in maintenance of the acid-base balance of the blood and tissues. Amino acids have both acid and base properties, enabling proteins to unite with either acid or alkaline substances in the blood and tissues. The reaction of blood and tissues normally is maintained as very slightly alkaline (ph 7.4) by a balance among several different factors, one of which is their respective protein content. Protein in the blood helps to prevent the accumulation of either too much base or too much acid in the blood and tissues.

Proteins also serve as chemical regulators of the body by helping to form substances in the blood called *antibodies,* which fight infection and infectious diseases.

4. To Activate Body Processes

Some proteins, called *enzymes* and *hormones*, are process-activators in making food available for use by the body.

Since food cannot be utilized directly by our bodies because the protein molecules are too large to pass through the fine pores in the intestinal wall, the food we eat must be "broken down" into amino acids. Part of the work is done by the process we know as digestion, the mechanical churning in the presence of strong stomach acid. But most of the "breaking down" is done by enzymes, the globular forms of protein that initiate and speed up chemical reactions within the cells.

Enzymes comprise the greatest number of all the proteins we make. Each cell makes untold hundreds of enzymes; they are present in the fluids of all cells. Each enzyme has unique characteristics that enable it to break down only one particular kind of protein. If one does not have a needed enzyme for a life process, the consequences to one's health can be serious.

Enzymes are shaped like pieces from a jigsaw puzzle, which enables them to interlock with specific proteins. By a method not fully understood, the enzyme snaps the protein apart into small amino acid molecules. These smaller molecules are able to pass through the walls of the intestine by a process called osmosis so they can be carried by the blood to the tissues. Each tissue utilizes specific amino acids by reassembling the various elements required to build its own characteristic proteins.

The other type of process-activating protein is hormones, protein substances secreted into the body from the endocrine glands. Hormones control and regulate the functions of various body processes, including the metabolism of carbohydrates, fats, and proteins. Also, hormones are important "message senders" in the body. The variety of hormones is almost beyond counting and their messages vary greatly, but the demands of hormones are largely for protein manufacture or breakdown. Each demand calls for the building blocks of life, primarily amino acids, and for fuel to do the work needed. Our food choices are, indirectly, responses to such demands.

The rate at which cells oxidize food is under the control of the thyroid gland. Thyroxine, the iodine-containing hormone secreted by the thyroid, regulates the oxidative processes by which body fuel is burned and energy set free. The internal secretion produced by the adrenals, two small glands situated just above the kidneys, and the insulin secreted by the pancreas are all especially important to the success of the athlete.

5. To Provide Body Energy

It is especially important to an athlete that the diet supply sufficient carbohydrate and fat foods to meet energy needs whenever new tissues are being formed. When energy needs from fats and carbohydrates are inadequate, proteins will provide the energy. If the total calorie count needed is not met, some of the proteins that should be allocated to building and repairing, regulating cell water and acid-base balances, and developing enzymes, antibodies, and hormones will be diverted from those functions to provide energy for the body's activities. Energy needs have a higher priority than maintenance of some tissue proteins; consequently, building or repairing processes will suffer.

Nitrogen, which is indispensable when protein is used for tissue building, is wasted when it is necessary to use protein for energy. The nitrogen-containing substances (chiefly urea) are excreted by the kidneys thus increasing their work. The rest of the protein is then oxidized in the same way that carbohydrates and fats are metabolized. Since energy is most economically supplied by carbohydrates and fats, the consumption of protein for energy is poor economy.

6. To Aid in Body Movements

Some proteins, called contractile proteins, actually can change shape; they can lengthen and shorten and thus make possible internal body movements as well as locomotion. Internal body movements include breathing, swallowing, the beating of the heart, and even the contracting of the stomach in hunger and in the actual digestive process.

The most active and abundant tissues of the body—the muscles and glandular organs—are high in protein content. Lean muscle, heart, and liver contain 17 to 21 percent protein. Protein compounds make up the contractile elements of all muscle fiber.

7. To Transport Body Materials

Transport proteins serve to carry things about in the body and deliver needed materials to the cells. The most familiar example is the hemoglobin of blood, which takes oxygen from the lungs to every part of the body, even the remotest extremity, so that fuel can be converted to energy.

STORING PROTEIN

Whether or not the body can build true protein reserves is

uncertain, but with a liberal protein intake, such tissues as the liver and muscles might have a slightly higher content of protein, amino acids, and other nitrogeneous products. This may constitute a small reserve that could be drawn on in time of protein lack or extra need.

DEFICIENCY OF PROTEIN

The effects of a diet deficient in protein might not be obvious for some time. Those who exist on a low-protein diet usually have less vitality and slower mental reactions. Their resistance to disease is also lower. They show signs of old age earlier than those who live on more adequate protein diets. One effect of an insufficient supply of protein is the development of a certain type of edema. The principal symptom of this disease is an excessive amount of water in the tissues. The liver is most susceptible to depletion of cellular protein, the muscles are relatively easy to deplete, and the brain is the most difficult.

Lysine, tryptophan, methionine, and thrionine are amino acids more likely to be deficient when people eat only cereal grains or legumes in very small amounts.

SUMMARY

Protein is the most complex substance known to man. It contains the life-sustaining element, nitrogen, combined in a complex organic compound. Man and animals cannot manufacture proteins but must obtain them ready-made from other animals and plants. Only plants can utilize the nitrogen in the soil to make protein. The building blocks of proteins are amino acids. Eight of them cannot be made in the human body and are called "essential" amino acids because they must be ingested in the diet; twelve amino acids can be synthesized in the body and are called "nonessential" because they need not be included in the diet although they are just as necessary for proper body functions. The body breaks proteins down into simple amino acids and then recombines them into new molecules. The number of combinations is nearly infinite.

Proteins differ greatly in food value, depending upon their amino acid composition. Proteins that contain all eight essential amino acids are called complete proteins, and generally they come from animal sources. All other proteins are incomplete proteins, and generally they come from plants. Incomplete protein foods should be combined with foods having complete proteins to make up for their deficiencies.

The principal functions of proteins are: to build new tissues, maintain and repair tissues, regulate body functions, activate and control body processes with enzymes and hormones, provide energy when there is a shortage of calories available, aid in body movements, and transport materials in the body.

Proteins can be stored in small amounts. A protein deficiency may result from a vegetarian diet, but that can be avoided easily. To build a body and keep it healthy, we must have a continuing supply of protein foods.

5

Vitamins—for Vim

The word "vitamin" comes from the Latin *vita,* meaning life. Vitamins are needed in tiny amounts by all living things; they sometimes are called the spark plugs of the human machine. Vitamins were identified early in this century when scientists realized that there are other essential substances in food besides proteins, carbohydrates, and fats.

Vitamins are not really food; they are merely chemical aids that the body uses to put food to work. They are necessary for healthy maintenance and growth. If vitamins are lacking in the diet, poor health or disease results.

Some plants can manufacture their own vitamins, but humans must get them from food (or other outside sources) since they cannot be manufactured by the body in required amounts.

Scientists have discovered about twenty-five different vitamins, although the exact function of each has not been determined. Upon discovery, researchers gave alphabet-letter names to the vitamins. At that time, they thought there were very few of these micronutrients. However, today there are nine vitamins designated as "B" vitamins, and the "B" designation means very little except that they are all water soluble and contain nitrogen.

Each of the nine "Bs" is a separate vitamin with unique functions, and each is found in varying proportions in different foods. The "Bs" have been given additional names such as "thiamin" for vitamin B-1 and "riboflavin" for vitamin B-2. Vitamin C is water soluble also and might be classed with the B-complex grouping except that it has no nitrogen.

Scientists divide vitamins into two general classes—those that dissolve in fat and those that dissolve in water. The water-soluble vitamins, such as those of the B-complex and vitamin C, are not stored in the body, so they must be included in the diet each day. They are thought to be safe in any quantity because the body merely excretes any excess amount taken. Thus the expression, "Excess vitamins, expensive urine"!

The fat-soluble group includes vitamins A, D, E, and K. These vitamins are associated with fatty foods such as butter, cream, vegetable oils, and the fats of meat and fish. Vitamin A also has been found in green leafy vegetables, which complicates understanding the sources of this vitamin.

Because fat-soluble vitamins can be stored in the body, principally in the liver, toxicity can develop if too great an amount of vitamin A or D is eaten. The excess cannot be excreted in the urine, as is the case with water-soluble vitamins. Vitamins A and D should be included in meals throughout the week but not necessarily every day. The fat-soluble vitamins, A, D, and E, are measured in International Units (IU) while the water-soluble vitamins are measured in milligrams (mg) or micrograms (mcg). Since care should be exercised in the amount of vitamins one consumes, read labels to be sure *what* and *how* much you consume.

Vitamin A, several B-complex vitamins, and vitamin C are commonly omitted in the diet. We don't eat enough fruits and vegetables to supply us with sufficient vitamins A and C. Important B vitamins are found in breads and cereals; but because we sometimes try to control our weight, we often omit bread, thinking that it is starchy and full of calories.

If we meet the vitamin requirements of A, B-1, B-2, C, and D in daily eating, we usually will have enough of all the other vitamins and minerals also.

Care should be taken in the preparation of foods to retain as many vitamins as possible. Vitamins are lost when fresh foods are not refrigerated, when foods are overcooked, when vegetables are processed in water and the liquid thrown away, and when soda is added to the vegetable water. Canned and frozen vegetables are about equal in vitamin content if the liquid is served and not thrown away.

Good food is the simplest and best way to be assured of the good health that nutrition can provide. Let us examine, then, what micronutrients we need as a way of learning which sources of protein, fat, and carbohydrate provide most completely for our needs.

VITAMIN A

Vitamin A is probably the most important of all vitamins—if we were to single out just one. Vitamin A occurs only in foods of animal origin, such as meat and dairy products, but also the body is able to form vitamin A from a pigment called carotene, which is present in deep yellow and dark green plant foods. Carotene gives a characteristic color to carrots, pumpkins, apricots, nectarines, corn, butter, cheddar cheese, and egg yolk. Carotene is used to color as well as to enrich margarines. Dark green vegetables also contain carotene; good vegetable vitamin A sources are broccoli, spinach, asparagus, and dark green lettuce. Usually, the deeper the color, the more vitamin A. The red of the tomato also contains the carotene color.

Function: Vitamin A is essential for growth, for the normal functioning of the eyes, especially in dim light, for the maintenance of clear, smooth skin, and for keeping the lining of mouth, nose, throat, and digestive tract healthy and disease-resistant.

Vitamin A also is essential for proper formation and maintenance of tooth enamel and the health of gums.

Sources: Since it is widely distributed in common foods, there is little reason for not getting all the vitamin A needed.

When more vitamin A is consumed than needed, the excess is stored in the liver. Because of this, animal livers are the richest source of A. One serving of calf's liver will supply all the vitamin A an adult needs for nearly a week. Fish-liver oils are also very rich sources of this vitamin.

One-half cup of spinach will provide two times as much vitamin A as the recommended daily allowance. Nutritionists recommend an occasional serving of super-rich A foods for storage purposes; eating liver every couple of weeks is a good habit.

Vitamin A and carotene are heat-resistant and aren't lost in processing, but they are destroyed by long contact with air through the process called oxidation.

Recommended Allowance: The recommended allowance for an adult is 5,000 IU each day; children require a little less. There are many myths about extra vitamin A improving resistance to infection. But once we have our 5,000 daily IU in good food, no additional amount will keep us from catching cold, and massive doses of vitamin A will not improve our eyesight beyond its natural potential. In general, supplements of this vitamin should be unnecessary.

How much vitamin A is toxic? The American Medical Association cautions that daily doses in excess of 50,000 IU can cause serious illness.

VITAMIN D

Vitamin D, the "sunshine vitamin," is the one vitamin that is hard to get enough of in ordinary foods unless the food is fortified. With the aid of sunshine, the body can synthesize its own vitamin D, and with just moderate exposure to sunlight the body seems to provide the vitamin D needs of most adults.

Function: Vitamin D helps the body use calcium and phosphorus, and in recent years the use of vitamin D milk and vitamin D concentrates for infants and children have greatly reduced the number of cases of rickets, a bone disease of small children.

Sources: The best food source of vitamin D is fortified milk and margarine. Other food sources include liver, the liver oil of saltwater fish, saltwater fish, egg yolks, and butter.

Vitamin D can be added to a number of foods by exposing them to ultraviolet rays in a light similar to sunlight. This process is called irradiation. Foods treated in this way are given such names as "vitamin D milk" and "irradiated evaporated milk." Fluid whole milk, skim milk, and evaporated milk are fortified with 400 units of vitamin D per quart.

Recommended Allowance: The dietary requirement of vitamin D for children is 400 IU. There is no dietary requirement for mature people, but it is suggested that they have a daily intake of about 400 IU. Most adults get all they need through diet and daily exposure to sunlight, but milk fortified with vitamin D is recommended for children because of its role in bone formation. Women should get a large amount of vitamin D during the months before childbirth.

Warning: Many food manufacturers are adding vitamin D to such foods as breakfast cereals, fruit drinks, candy, etc. This is an advertising scheme to make the product sound especially good, but excess vitamin D stored in the body could be a health problem if the amount stored is high enough to create a toxicity situation. When in doubt, check the label for vitamin D amounts.

VITAMIN E

Vitamin E has been called the "rejuvenation vitamin." Vitamin E is considered necessary to human development although only a very small amount is needed. Vitamin E is known as the vitamin searching for a disease!

Function: Its chief function is thought to be as an antioxidant. An antioxidant inhibits the combination of a substance with oxygen and thus acts as a preservative. Vitamin E protects vitamin A and carotene from destruction by oxidation.

Vitamin E was first believed to prevent sterility, and it is erroneously believed to have vast curative powers, but, as yet, none of these claims has been proven. There is no evidence that vitamin E supplements increase the strength and endurance of athletes. There might be a psychological effect, but that is all.

Vitamin E is necessary in the diet, but there is no scientific evidence that it will do any of the dramatic things claimed for it. Sales have soared for vitamin E supplements even though no need for these products has been proven.

Sources: Vitamin E is available in adequate quantities in the ordinary diet. It is supplied in substantial amounts in vegetable oils as well as margarine and shortening made from these oils. Wheat germ oil is a rich source. Other sources are green leafy vegetables, whole grain cereals, meat, egg yolk, fish, and liver; also legumes, nuts, and poultry.

Recommended Allowance: The Recommended Dietary Allowance (RDA) for vitamin E is set at 4-5 IU for infants, 7-12 IU for children, and 12-15 IU for men and women.

As we increase our consumption of polyunsaturated fats in order to lower cholesterol, we should also increase, proportionally, our consumption of vitamin E foods.

Caution: Vitamin E in large doses appears to affect calcium absorption in the body, lowers thyroid output, and limits the uptake of vitamin K from the intestine. Too much vitamin E can cause hemorrhages in the skin.

VITAMIN K

Vitamin K is a fat-soluble, yellow vitamin that is essential for proper coagulation of blood. The designation "K" derives from the German *koagulation.* Vitamin K appears not to be useful to the body other than in its role in clotting.

Function: The primary function of vitamin K in the body is the formation in the liver of a protein called prothrombin, which is necessary for clotting, or coagulation. Prothrombin is converted to its active form, thrombin, which is necessary for the formation of fibrin, a protein that is the basis for blood clots. Without vitamin K, prothrombin cannot be formed, and blood will not clot.

The athlete prone to injury or facing surgery should be aware of the importance of this vitamin to his particular state of health.

Sources: Vitamin K is plentiful in all green leafy vegetables, liver, egg yolks, soybean oil, cauliflower, and especially the outer leaves of cabbage. Little vitamin K is present in animal products.

Vitamin K is quite stable to heat, air, and moisture but not to light. Cooking destroys very little of the vitamin because it is not water soluble.

With a normal diet, an adequate amount of vitamin K is manufactured in the body due to the bacteria present in the human intestinal tract. This source provides considerable vitamin K for most persons.

Recommended Allowance: The adult minimum requirement for this vitamin is thought to be around 30 mcg per day since that amount was necessary to restore clotting in a group of vitamin K-depleted adults. This vitamin is among the most potent of all the vitamins. No allowance for vitamin K has been set by the Food and Nutrition Board. The layman need give vitamin K very little thought.

Vitamin K has proved ineffective in hemophilia, an inherited condition causing hemorrhaging in man.

VITAMIN C

Vitamin C is a water-soluble vitamin called the "orange juice vitamin." It also is known as ascorbic acid, an essential food substance needed to prevent scurvy. Almost all animals are able to produce it from sugars within their own bodies, but man must depend on his supply of the vitamin from his food.

Function: Vitamin C is required in the metabolism of many substances in the body. Just how or why vitamin C is associated with so many and such varied chemical changes that are part of normal metabolism in the tissues is not yet known, but enough is known to establish it as a very important substance for body welfare.

One of the most important functions of vitamin C is its role in the production of collagen, a substance that binds cells together and keeps them in proper relation to each other. Vitamin C also helps in the maintenance of the capillary blood vessels, and it is an aid in healing wounds. Vitamin C influences the formation of hemoglobin, the absorption of iron from the intestine, and deposition of iron in liver tissue. It also takes part in a number of reactions involving the vitamin folacin and amino acids such as tyrosine and tryptophan.

Vitamin C is involved in the chemical synthesis of the adrenal gland hormones. One of these, adrenalin, helps release glycogen reserves from the liver into the blood as glucose, which greatly enhances energy levels in training and competition. Vitamin C helps in removal of lactic acid, the waste product of carbohydrate metabolism. The vitamin is important also in prevention of muscular weakness and in the development of strong bones, sound teeth, and firm gums. Vitamin C also functions in some little-understood way in protecting the body against infections and bacterial toxins. Infections apparently decrease the amount of ascorbic acid in tissues and body fluids.

Sources: Vitamin C is present in oranges, lemons, limes, green peppers, grapefruit, strawberries, raw cabbage, salad greens, and tomatoes. Baked and boiled potatoes are also good sources of this vitamin. Vitamin C is the most easily destroyed of all vitamins. Foods containing vitamin C should be eaten raw whenever possible in order to maintain their maximum vitamin content. Since vitamin C is water soluble and thus cannot be stored, it should be replenished daily.

Good foods should be used as the source of vitamin C; there

is no need for supplements unless the doctor orders them. The vitamin also can be obtained in pure form under the generic name ascorbic acid.

Many experiments with human volunteers indicate that the body has wide tolerances for vitamin C lacks and excesses. One of the signs of a deficiency of vitamin C is greater susceptiblity to infection. This has led to the belief that vitamin C is a curative or preventive for colds and other assorted illnesses.

Extra Amounts: Dr. Linus Pauling, Nobel-prize winning chemist, recommends taking one or two grams of ascorbic acid a day to prevent colds. That is twenty to forty times the average adult need, and he urges that one raise this to four grams a day if catching a cold.

In the past few years there have been numerous studies on the effect of vitamin C as an aid in the prevention and reduction of common cold symptoms. Linus Pauling might be correct in his theory that megadoses of vitamin C (one to four grams per day) will prevent or reduce the symptoms of common viral ailments, especially the cold. Vitamin C *may* be beneficial in reducing the severity of colds or reducing the length of time that symptoms persist, but findings do not indicate positive proof nor do they indicate that Vitamin C can prevent the occurrence of colds.

Vitamin C taken in food is absorbed into the bloodstream chiefly from the small intestine within a few hours after it is ingested. The level of vitamin C in blood plasma is increased only temporarily because this substance is taken up by the tissues. The body uses only the amount of ascorbic acid it needs and eliminates the rest through the kidneys. When body tissues are saturated with vitamin C, additional intake is excreted in the urine. But when body tissues are depleted of vitamin C, a high intake is absorbed and retained. There is no evidence that amounts greatly in excess of normal, recommended intake confer extra benefits except after deprivation or during periods of unusual physical stress.

Recommended Allowance: 40 to 55 mg for children; 45 mg for women; 60 mg for men.

Heavy smokers have lowered blood levels of vitamin C and

an apparent increased requirement, but this is well within the range of the recommended allowance. No increased demand for vitamin C has been reported for elderly people, but under certain conditions of continued stress and drug therapy there may be need for an increased amount of the vitamin.

TABLE 5-1   FOODS CONTAINING VITAMIN C*

Vegetable Source	Amount	Milligrams of Vitamin C
Kale (cooked)	1/2 cup	93
Broccoli	1/2 cup	62
Green pepper	1 small	60
Turnip greens (cooked)	1/2 cup	52
Brussel sprouts	4 average	40
Cauliflower	1/2 cup	40
Tomato (raw)	1 medium	35
Asparagus (cooked)	6 stalks	26
Spinach (cooked)	1/2 cup	25
Sweet potato (baked)	1 medium	22
Cabbage	1/2 cup	21
Tomato juice	1/2 cup	20
Lettuce	4 large dark green leaves	20
Potato, white baked	1 medium	16
Green peas (cooked)	1/2 cup	16
Squash, winter (cooked)	1/2 cup	10
Fruit Source		
Orange juice	1/2 cup	62
Strawberries	1/2 cup	45
Grapefruit	one-half	44
Grapefruit juice	1/2 cup	42
Cantaloupe, slice	4 ounces	33
Cantaloupe, cubes	1/2 cup	33
Banana	1 medium	12
Apricots (raw)	2-3 medium	10
Peach (raw)	1 medium	8
Apple (raw)	1 large	7
Watermelon, slice	4 ounces	7
Watermelon, cubes	1/2 cup	7

* Figures are from U.S. Department of Agriculture No. 8, *Composition of Foods Raw, Processed, Prepared*, approved for reprinting October, 1975.

Millions of Americans are dosing themselves with *extra* vitamin C—usually in amounts of 100 mg per day, almost twice the daily recommended need. The practice is not known to be dangerous, but to nutritionists it just doesn't make sense.

Caution: Excessive doses might pose serious hazards! Anyone ingesting large (0.5 gm or more) doses of vitamin C daily should have an evaluation of vitamin B-12. It has been shown that large doses of vitamin C actually destroy vitamin B-12.

VITAMIN B-COMPLEX

The vitamins of the vitamin B-complex usually are classed together because they were first thought to be a single vitamin, which was named vitamin B. Then scientists found that this substance was composed of several vitamins, all water soluble.

So far, nine vitamins have been "discovered" in the B-complex; some are better known than others. Although all B vitamins have distinctive properties and, hence, will be described separately, they are intimately interrelated in the body's cellular reactions.

The "big three" of B vitamins are thiamin (B-1), riboflavin (B-2), and niacin (sometimes incorrectly called B-3). These three vitamins are involved primarily in the release of energy. Heavy exercise and athletic training require an increased intake of foods containing the B-complex vitamins: thiamin, riboflavin, niacin, and also pantothenic acid.

One protection against dietary deficiencies of the B-vitamin "big three" is the enrichment of flours. But not all bread is enriched, and many other grain products needlessly lack enrichment, among them cakes, cookies, pastries, etc. It is important to read the labels of all flour products and to watch for the adjective "enriched" in the contents. Nutritionists see no excuse for omitting enrichment. It is a cheap and simple safety measure and acceptable for good nutrition.

A diet high in proteins as well as fruits and vegetables generally insures against a deficiency of these vitamins.

Enriched breakfast cereals and enriched breads contribute significantly to daily requirements of thiamin, riboflavin, and niacin. In addition to B vitamins, whole-grain bread contains many other vitamins and minerals as well.

There appear to be no other B vitamins than the nine although many compounds are being studied in various laboratories, and these are conveniently termed "unidentified factors." It remains to be seen whether any of these "unidentified factors" turn out to be B vitamins or whether they are needed by man.

Many natural, organic "growth factors" other than vitamins are necessary for lower forms of life. These include nucleic acids, purines and pyrimidines, peptides, sterols, and others, none of which fit the definition of a vitamin.

If one eats a variety of foods from the basic four food groups (which supply ample amounts of all the B vitamins), there should be no cause for concern.

Vitamin B-1, Thiamin

Thiamin sometimes is called the "pep vitamin" or the "morale vitamin" since people who do not get enough thiamin feel tired, irritable, and depressed. Thiamin also has been called the "appetite vitamin" because a deficiency causes loss of appetite. The "thio" of thiamin means sulfur-containing. Thiamin is a crystalline substance made of carbon, hydrogen, oxygen, and sulfur. It is readily soluble in water.

Function: Thiamin plays a part in promoting appetite and better functioning of the digestive tract, effects that have an indirect influence in promoting growth.

Thiamine is needed as a co-enzyme in the processes of getting oxygen to body tissues, using carbohydrates, and building ribose, the sugar that is such an important part of cell structure. Thiamin is needed also for proper functioning of the heart. Vitamin B-1 is the substance that prevents or cures beriberi, a disorder of the nervous system.

Sources: In plants thiamin is concentrated chiefly in seeds (whole grains, legumes, and nuts); in animals it is abundant in the organs (liver, heart, kidneys). Pork flesh is much higher in thiamin content than other meats, but meats and leafy vegetables are moderately good sources. Such foods as oatmeal and dried legumes can be economical sources of thiamin. Breads and cereals of moderate thiamin content should be enriched with the synthetic vitamin.

Our best sources of thiamin—whole grains, organ meats, pork, and legumes—are not used in quantity by the American people.

Recommended Allowance: Allowances for thiamin usually are related to energy intake. A thiamin allowance of 0.5 mg/1,000 calories is recommended for all ages. Thiamin deficiency often occurs in adults. Since thiamin is water soluble, it cannot be stored in the body, and the amount of the vitamin not required for day-to-day use is excreted in the urine.

Vitamin B-2, Riboflavin

Vitamin B-2 was formerly known as vitamin B or G. It has been called the "anti-old-age vitamin" because a diet rich in riboflavin helps protect against disease and seems to prevent too rapid aging.

Function: The chief function of riboflavin is the role it plays in the metabolism of carbohydrate, protein, and fat. During this process, energy is released and made available to the cells for growth and repair of the body.

Riboflavin is part of several enzymes and co-enzymes that enter into many body-chemistry processes. It is especially noteworthy as a carrier of hydrogen and for promoting the body's use of oxygen. Riboflavin is essential for good health and proper growth. It is necessary for the health of the skin and the proper functioning of the eyes in adjusting to intensity of light.

Sources: Riboflavin is widely distributed in both plant and animal tissues. Milk, cheese, eggs, liver and other organ meats, lean meats, fish, poultry, legumes, bread, dried yeast, and leafy vegetables are foods among the richest in riboflavin. Milk is the best dietary source of riboflavin. Milk has about four times more riboflavin than thiamin while the whole-grain cereals, which are among the richest sources of thiamin, have only a moderate amount of riboflavin.

Like thiamin, riboflavin can be dissolved in cooking water; save the water in which the foods are cooked, and use it in soups or in creaming vegetables. Riboflavin is heat-resistant but destroyed by sunlight. Sunlight striking milk in glass bottles can destroy over half of the riboflavin in a couple of hours. It is best to keep milk in a cool, dark place, such as a refrigerator, as much of the time as possible.

Recommended Allowance: The amount of riboflavin needed is related to body size, metabolic rate, and rapidity of growth. The recommended allowance for males 11-22 years of age is 1.5 to 1.8 mg and for females 11-22 years of age, 1.3-1.4 mg. There does not appear to be any specialized mechanism for storage of riboflavin. Unused riboflavin is excreted in the urine.

Niacin

Niacin, the third member of the vitamin B-complex, is called the "anti-pellagra" vitamin. Niacin also is called nicotinic acid (not to be confused with nicotine). Nicotinic acid and the related compound nicotinamide are white compounds, soluble in water, and stable to both heating and oxidation as well as to acids and alkalis.n

Function: Niacin is present in two important co-enzymes that are essential in the process of oxidation-reduction reactions. One enzyme assists in oxidizing lactic acid in the tissues and another is essential in the formation of water. Lack of niacin to form these co-enzymes in sufficient quantities handicaps vital chemical processes and may result in injury to tissues throughout the body. Niacin is also important in promoting growth, proper functioning of the nervous system, and a generally good physical and mental state of health—free from depression.

Sources: Most foods that are good sources of thiamin and riboflavin, namely, organ meats such as liver, lean meats, fish (especially tuna and salmon), whole grains, yeast, legumes, nuts, peanuts, and wheat germ, are also high in niacin content.

Niacin can be synthesized by bacteria in the intestine, and it can be made in the tissues from the amino acid tryptophan. Niacin is heat-resistant; little is lost in cooking unless the cooking water is discarded.

The cost of enrichment of foods with niacin is negligible. Niacin is so inexpensive and so readily available in our foods that pellagra should be a disease of the past.

Recommended Allowance: The requirement for niacin varies with the nature of the diet, that is, whether the protein furnishes much or little tryptophan. Approximately 1 mg of niacin may be expected to be formed for each 60 mg of tryptophan in the diet.

Amount needed: Males 11-22 years old need 18-20 mg; females 11-22 years old need 14-16 mg. A riboflavin-deficient diet usually will be a niacin-deficient one as well.

Vitamin B-6, Pyridoxine

Pyridoxine is probably the form you see most on labels, and it is largely of *vegetable* origin; pyridoxal and pyridoxamine are the other two B-6 chemicals, and they occur mainly in *animal* products. Any of these serve as the vitamin. Whichever type is consumed, the body uses it as the raw material for making a chemical called pyridoxal phosphate. This is a co-enzyme and a basic body tool.

Function: B-6, or pyridoxine, is necessary for protein and fat metabolism and affects muscular control; it is essential to development of the nervous system in infants; and it helps protect the health of red blood cells, the nervous system, and the skin.

B-6 contributes to good mental health. Like all the B vitamins, pyridoxine is essential for normal functioning of the central nervous system and the transmission of brain impulses. So far, some two dozen amino-acid reactions are known to require B-6. Obviously, without this vitamin we do not operate very well.

Sources: Vitamin B-6 follows the general distribution of most other B vitamins. The best sources are meats (especially liver), some vegetables (including potatoes), wheat germ, wheat bran, whole-grain cereals, yeast, soybeans, and sunflower seeds. In milling white flour more than 75 percent of the vitamin B-6 content of wheat is lost; it is not added in the enrichment programs although there are good arguments for doing so. Synthetic pyridoxine is quite inexpensive.

Recommended Allowance: For males 11-22 and older, 1.6-2.0 mg per day. For females 11-22 and older, 1.6-2.0 mg per day. The body's needs are so small that deficiencies are rare.

Folacin

Folacin, the generic term for folic acid and related compounds, is one of the most important vitamins. Sometimes known as folate, (formerly, just folic acid) this B vitamin gets its name from *folium,* the Latin word for foliage or leaf, because it was first isolated from spinach leaves and was known to be widely distributed in green leafy plants.

Function: Folacin aids in protein metabolism, contributes to normal growth and reproduction, and is essential for the formation and development to maturity of red blood cells. The consequences of an inadequate supply can be serious. Although all animals require folacin, some species can meet this need by the production of the vitamin through bacterial synthesis in the intestine. Man must have folacin supplied in the food in order to avoid deficiency symptoms.

Sources: Meats are poor sources of folic acid; leaves are best! The richest sources are liver, yeast, and leafy vegetables. Good sources are dried legumes, green vegetables (such as asparagus, deep green lettuce, and broccoli), nuts, fresh oranges, and whole wheat products. The choice of at least one serving of green leafy vegetables per day should contribute significantly to meeting the daily requirements of folacin.

The use of synthetic folacin in vitamin supplements or for food enrichment has certain legal restrictions, so it is important to depend on dietary sources for normal supply.

Recommended Allowance: A total of 0.4 mg per day of folacin activity is recommended for adult men and women. This is higher than previous estimates but takes into account possible losses from cooking, poor absorption, and varying activity of the several forms of folacin in foods.

Vitamin B-12, Cobalamin

Vitamin B-12, the "miracle" or "red" vitamin, known as cobalamin, was the last vitamin to be discovered in the B-complex vitamin grouping. Distinguishing characteristics are its red color, the presence in its molecule of cobalt and phosphorus, and (unlike any other vitamin) the inability of higher plants to synthesize it. Vitamin B-12 is another very basic element of cell survival, but it is another vitamin that poses no problems for most of us.

Function: Vitamin B-12 is involved in the development of red blood cells and is effective in the prevention as well as treatment of pernicious anemia. It also is involved in the making of nucleic and amino acids and in the workings of the nervous system and digestive tract. The role of vitamin B-12 in metabolism is not completely understood, but it is essential for the normal functioning of all body cells.

Sources: Animal products are the primary dietary sources of B-12. Richest sources are liver and organ meats. Muscle meats, fish, eggs, shellfish, milk, and most milk products except butter are good sources.

Grains, vegetables, and fruits have trace amounts that are absorbed from the B-12 vitamin-rich soil while the plant is growing. There is none present in yeast, the traditional source of other B-complex vitamins, but some special yeasts containing vitamin B-12 are available. They have been grown on media very rich in the vitamin, which is then absorbed in the yeast cell.

Vitamin B-12 is the most complicated of all the vitamins and the only one that chemists have not yet learned to synthesize in the laboratory. Fortunately, highly active vitamin B-12 concentrates can be produced inexpensively by the vitamin industry from cultures of certain bacteria and fungi grown in large tanks containing special media. These concentrates, universally used as the source of B-12 in vitamin supplements, have not been used to enrich man's food. (One year's supply for one normal person costs about two cents.)

Vitamin B-12 promises to be one of the most important vitamins for mankind. It is now possible to use plant and cereal foods much more wisely in the human diet in case of future population pressures, famines, or during periods when animal foods are in short supply.

Recommended Allowance: If absorption is normal, a dietary intake of three micrograms per day of vitamin B-12 is required for both sexes from youth to old age to ensure the replacement of normal losses.

The Food and Nutrition Board finds that average American diets meet these requirements quite adequately. There is a possible exception, however: the group of vegetarians who do not eat milk, eggs, cheese, or fish.

Pantothenic Acid

Pantothenic acid, a member of the B-complex, was given this Greek title meaning "from everything." Pantothenic acid is a part of co-enzyme A, where it is essential for the synthesis, breakdown, and release of energy from carbohydrates, fats, and proteins. Thus, every cell gets its energy and some of its basic building blocks of carbons, hydrogens, and oxygens. Since all foods ultimately require pantothenic acid to be converted to energy, this vitamin is one of the most important substances in body metabolism.

Function: Pantothenic acid is needed for the formation of such important sterols as cholesterol and the adrenocortical hormones. It functions also as a component of the enzyme involved in the synthesis of acetylcholine, an important regulator of nerve tissue.

Because of its role of building many essential complicated compounds out of simpler ones, pantothenic acid is a dietary essential for man.

Sources: Pantothenic acid is found in *all* living cells, plant and animal, and therefore is present in all natural foods. It is widely distributed in foods of animal origin and also in whole grains and legumes.

The foods with the most pantothenic acid include yeast, eggs, liver, kidney, peanuts, dried peas, and the germs and bran of wheat and rice. Processing and refinement of foods can result in considerable loss of pantothenic acid.

Recommended Allowance: The dietary requirement of pantothenic acid for man is unknown, but the Food and Nutrition Board has suggested that 5 to 10 mg per day is adequate for children and adults (a recommended allowance has not been set).

Synthetic calcium pantothenate is widely used today, though usually only in trivial amounts, in vitamin supplements and to fortify a few breakfast foods.

Biotin

Biotin, a member of the vitamin B-complex, is a water-soluble compound widely distributed in nature. It is one of the lesser known vitamins of the B-complex. An early name for it was the "anti-egg white injury factor." It contains sulfur in its chemical formula.

Biotin, like pantothenic acid, was known to be a growth factor for yeast before its vitamin nature was discovered. It was given the name "biotin" because it was part of the *bios* factor needed for yeast growth. In foods and animal tissues it is bound to protein.

Function: Biotin is involved with making fatty acids, with the food-energy cycles in the production of energy from glucose, in making glycogen to store energy in the liver, and in amino acid building.

Most biotin in the body is combined in various enzymes by means of chemical union with the amino acid lysine. These reactions are closely involved with those of pantothenic acid.

Sources: It is widely distributed in foods known to be good sources of the other B-complex vitamins. Yeast, egg yolk, and liver are exceptionally good sources.

We have two protections against biotin deficiency. One is the fact that there is plenty of this vitamin in the foods we eat, and, in addition, the bacteria living in our intestines make enough biotin to supply our requirements, usually with some to spare. There is a special protein called avidin in raw egg white that combines with biotin in the intestinal tract, thus rendering the biotin unabsorbable. This so-called "egg-white injury" can be overcome eating biotin-rich food such as egg yolk, liver, or yeast.

It would be very rare to encounter biotin deficiency among humans unless a person consumes large amounts of raw eggs (eight to ten per day) without extra biotin sources. However, the occasional eating of a few eggs, as in eggnog, does not provide sufficient avidin to produce biotin deficiency.

Recommended Allowance: There is no known figure for the requirement of biotin for man. The Food and Nutrition Board of the United States estimates that the average American diet supplies about 0.15 to 0.30 mg of biotin per day, which is sufficient to take care of human needs. Microorganisms in the intestinal tract of man synthesize large amounts of biotin.

It is interesting to note that three to six times more biotin is excreted in the urine than is ingested, reflecting the major contribution of intestinal bacteria.

We need not worry about a shortage of biotin unless we use heavy doses of antibiotics, but it is possible to kill off some of the friendly microbial biotin-makers and still have a sufficient supply because of the ease of getting biotin in ordinary food. The Food and Nutrition Board is quite sure that we get plenty.

Choline

Choline is an important vitamin in the B group, and it is used in larger quantities than any other vitamin substance. Because a vitamin is partly defined by identifying it with a deficiency, there has been uncertainty about designating choline as a vitamin. No one has been able to find a person suffering from choline deficiency.

However, a dietary requirement for choline can be demonstrated experimentally for at least ten species of animals, including the rat, dog, pig, and monkey. Thus, it is officially declared a vitamin.

Function: Choline (generally combined with other compounds) has several catalytic and metabolic functions in the body: as a constituent of several phospholipids (primarily lecithin), it aids in the transport and metabolism of fats; as a constituent of acetylocholine, it plays a role in normal functioning of the nervous system; also, it participates in the body's synthesis of proteins. It is essential for growth.

Choline prevents the accumulation of fat in the liver, a condition called "fatty liver" in animals.

Sources: Choline is present in fat-like substances called phospholipids, such as lecithin, and is very plentiful in egg yolk (probably the richest natural source), liver and other organ meats (such as kidney, heart, and brain), meats of all types, legumes, and wheat germ. Moderate amounts are found in milk and vegetables but very little in fruits.

Recommended Allowance: The Food and Nutrition Board has seen no point in suggesting even a tentative RDA for choline since the quantity synthesized by the body is not known and the requirement for choline is influenced not only by the amounts of methionine, folic acid, and vitamin B-12 in the diet but also by growth rate, energy intake and expenditure, fat intake, and the type of dietary fat.

Mixed diets are estimated to provide human adults with 400 to 900 mg of choline daily. Such amounts evidently are adequate. Ignore exaggerated claims made for choline-rich foods and chemicals, including lecithin.

INOSITOL

For a time, researchers thought inositol might be a B vitamin, but it is not. Inositol is a "growth factor" for certain yeasts.

Occasionally, it will be listed among the B-complex vitamins (on labels, catalogs, diet-ingredient lists, etc.)

Every once in a while, a health food promoter will rediscover inositol, probably saying it helps prevent hardening of the arteries. Ignore the promotion. Our own cells make all the inositol we need not to mention that it is available in the food we normally eat. Whole grains, nuts, fruits, and meats are good sources of inositol.

PABA, OR PARA-AMINOBENZOIC ACID

Another constituent of foods is para-aminobenzoic acid, often listed with the B vitamins. It is important as a "growth factor" for lower animals. It has no vitamin activity if animals receive ample folacin, and it is no longer considered a vitamin. PABA should not be listed in the B-vitamin group. Its natural source is yeast. It is promoted to cure fatigue and eczema.

VITAMIN P, THE NON-VITAMIN

In the 1930s some chemists thought they had discovered a "new" vitamin, which was found in certain fruits and other fruits. It sometimes was referred to as citrin. Claims were made, but they did not prove true. They are still being made, and they still are not true. By 1950 it was resolved that the term Vitamin P be abandoned.

This material, now called bioflavenoids, includes substances called hesperidin and rutin. They might have uses in the pharmaceutical industry. Although described commonly as nutrients, there is as yet no evidence that they are required by man or that they can lessen the need for vitamin C, as was once supposed.

6

Minerals—Your Gold Mine

Our body is an exceptional creation, made of inexpensive materials but designed to function with highest precision.

Non-metallic elements make up 96 percent of body weight. The remaining elements are minerals—not as a geologist thinks of minerals, but as elements making up different combinations in the body.

Mineral elements originate in the soil, with plants taking up the inorganic elements they need in their life processes. Man and animals eat the plants. In this way humans obtain the minerals they need by eating not only plants but also animal tissue and animal products. Thus, minerals of the soil become minerals of the body.

Minerals usually are separated into two groups: those that occur in the body and in foods in relatively *large* amounts (such as calcium, phosphorus, magnesium, potassium, sodium, and sulfur); and those that occur and are needed in *trace* amounts (iron, iodine, zinc, fluorine, cobalt, manganese, copper, chromium, molybdenum, selenium, vanadium, nickel, tin, etc.). All told, some 50 known minerals are thought to contribute to our health.

Of the trace elements we need only a few milligrams per day while our need is for 100 milligrams per day of those with more structural responsibilities. Although minerals are identified separately, they rarely act alone; they act together and in various combinations in a marvel of cooperative effort.

Minerals, as elements and as salts, have two general body functions: building and regulating. They are needed in body building to provide rigidity and strength to soft tissues, bones, and teeth. Regulating functions include such varied responsibilities as balance of body fluid, regularity of heart beat, nerve response, movement of oxygen from lungs to tissues, and blood clotting.

Minerals tend to be incorporated into the actual structure and functioning of chemicals in the body while vitamins serve in a catalytic way—as in digestion—without actually becoming part of the products of the reaction. However, minerals become involved in building enzymes, which then work as catalysts, and finally in building actual tissue structures such as bone and teeth.

There are a number of things we do not know about the function of minerals in the body—particularly the trace elements—but we are in awe of their tiny quantity and their overwhelming accomplishment. It should be emphasized that people who take mineral supplements should not use them in amounts greatly in excess of what the body requires. Mineral metabolism is extremely complex. A delicate natural balance could be disrupted.

The National Research Council has established recommended dietary allowances for calcium, phosphorus, magnesium, iron, iodine, and zinc. It is believed that if the requirements for these and other nutrients on the recommended table are met, the remaining minerals also will be present in adequate amounts.

A normal, well-balanced diet as the source of a sufficient

supply of all necessary vitamins and minerals cannot be emphasized enough!

CALCIUM

Calcium, a relatively inert element, is present in the body in greater amounts than any other mineral; it represents about 40 percent of the body's total mineral content. The largest part of the body's calcium is in the bones and teeth, with a very small amount (about 1 percent) contained in soft tissues, blood, and other body fluids.

Most of us have between two and three pounds of calcium in our body. We perhaps think of calcium in the bones as in a permanent state, but bones are constantly being formed and reabsorbed—rapidly during early development and at a declining rate during adult life. In an adult it has been estimated that about 700 mg of calcium enter and leave the bones each day. Inactivity or immobilization causes the bones to decalcify, and this can be a problem (or at least a consideration) for athletes with fractures or torn ligaments that prevent ambulation. The bones are about two-thirds mineral compounds and one-third protein substances. They are very much alive; consider the marvelous self-mending that bones are able to accomplish.

In the blood from one-third to one-half of the calcium is present as inorganic salts (chiefly phosphates or bicarbonates) and the remainder is combined with protein and acted upon by enzymes before use in metabolism.

Function: Although the amount of calcium in soft tissues is small compared with that in bones, its presence is essential and its concentration must be kept within very narrow limits for the body to function normally.

The teeth and bones cannot absorb calcium unless the diet contains a small amount of phosphorus. A supply of vitamin D also is necessary. The proper balance between calcium, sodium, potassium, and magnesium is necessary for normal rhythmic contraction and relaxation of the heart muscles.

Calcium in blood plasma is one of the essential factors for blood clotting; it markedly affects muscle tone and irritability; and it is required for normal nerve transmission.

Deficiency: Calcium is one of the minerals in which the diet is most likely to be deficient. An inadequate supply of calcium in the diet of adults may not become apparant for a long time. Its lack may cause a withdrawal of calcium from the bones and teeth; usually the withdrawal is from the bone ends, called trabeculae. Good, strong teeth are not affected immediately by a calcium shortage. Withdrawal of calcium may result in soft, porous bones, dental decay, and eventually rickets, a disease in which the bones are so soft that they become deformed. Such deformities can last a lifetime.

Sources: In the United States about three-fourths of the calcium intake is derived from milk and dairy products; milk and hard cheeses are excellent choices. In addition, dark green leafy vegetables (the dark green leaves of lettuce contain more calcium than the light green leaves) and soft fish bones (canned salmon, sardines, etc.) are rich sources. Soft cheeses, cottage cheese, legumes, nuts and grains, and fruits and vegetables contain some calcium. Most fruits and vegetables, bread, and breakfast cereals contain relatively minor amounts but if eaten in considerable quantities, may add appreciably to calcium intake.

Recommended Allowance: Inadequate dietary calcium is one of our primary nutritional concerns. The problem is especially acute among growing adolescents, including athletes, who need a good supply of calcium for bone growth as well as bone strengthening and repair. For the athlete, calcium requirements also are influenced by high levels of protein intake—the greater the protein intake, the greater the calcium loss.

In addition, the average daily loss of calcium in sweat is about 15 mg, and strenuous physical activity increases the loss—even during periods of low calcium intake. Vitamin D plays an important role in both the absorption and utilization of calcium. Calcium is required for normal assimilation of protein and phosphorus.

Absorption of calcium from the intestinal tract varies with different individuals and under different conditions, but it is not as complete as for some other nutrients. The relative amounts of calcium retained in the body vary, depending on the age of the person, his previous habits of calcium consumption, and the amount he currently is consuming. A higher proportion of calcium is utilized when intake is low than when it is liberal. Ingested calcium is absorbed incompletely from the gut, and normally, depending on the intake, 70 to 80 percent of the calcium in the diet is excreted in the feces.

For adults 800 mg per day of calcium is recommended. Adults need calcium only for maintenance of a body already built, but they require more calcium than once was thought necessary. For children from 2 to 5 years of age the calcium allowance is the same as for adults: 800 mg; 6 to 10 years, the allowance is 1,000 mg; 11 to 18 years, 1,200 mg.

Bone Growth: The team of calcium, phosphorous, protein, and vitamins C and D builds bones. Milk and milk products provide most of the calcium for good bone growth. When bones are growing, the weakest part is just above and below a joint such as the knee, ankle, elbow, or wrist and near the ends of ribs. This is where the growing layer is forming new bone.

Reasons for Calcium Lack: There is a tendency to refuse milk products because of cholesterol-heart-disease problems, but skim milk is available and good. Be sure to get skim milk fortified with vitamins A and D. Eating other good calcium sources such as nuts and legumes is being cut back, unfortunately, because of fear of overweight.

There is a growing decline in use of vegetables because more and more people frequent fast food services. What passes as a salad in many eating places is very pale lettuce indeed, so learn to make your own at home; remember to get the deepest green lettuce you can! Greenness is a good indicator of vitamin and mineral content.

Another reason for calcium lack is that more and more people are on vegetarian diets, and they are not getting a sufficient allowance of calcium. Adding a pint of milk or cheese makes an important calcium contribution to the diet.

Calcium Lactate: If calcium is taken in pill form (by doctor's advice), it should be in the form of some soluble salt such as calcium lactate. Unless there is some excellent reason (allergy to milk), it is far better to revise the diet to include more calcium-rich foods, which furnish, along with calcium, other minerals and vitamins that are important to the body.

Calcium exists in nature in such common substances as chalk, limestone, granite, egg shell, sea shells, "hard water," and bone (all of which can serve as a source of calcium in the diet if one wishes to incorporate them in some way.) Primitive man ate small bones—cracked them and chewed on them.

PHOSPHORUS

Phosphorus is the second most abundant mineral in man. About 80 percent of the phosphorus is in the bones and teeth while 20 percent of the phosphorus content of the body is present mostly in soft tissues, with some phosphorus in every cell. It is one of the most important nutrients known, taking part in almost every reaction in the body. Phosphorus, a nonmetallic element, exists in nature only in combined forms, usually with calcium.

Phosphorus is itself highly reactive and imparts this property to substances with which it is combined. Phosphorus is present in or combines readily with proteins, lipids, or carbohydrates. Chemically inert substances such as glucose and fats become highly reactive in tissue metabolism and more readily transported in body fluids by combination with phosphate (PO_4) radicals. Phosphorus is absorbed through the intestinal wall and carried by the blood in more soluble forms to all parts of the body. From one-half to two-thirds of the phosphorus in blood is contained within the red cells.

Functions: Phosphorus performs an important role in combining with calcium to give rigidity to bones and teeth (the presence of vitamin D also is essential).

Inorganic phosphates in the blood act as buffer substances

that assist in maintaining blood neutrality and the acid-base balance of the blood.

Phosphates are indispensable to the oxidation of carbohydrates, from which much of the energy for body processes is obtained. Phosphorus is vital to liberation of energy. It also helps control the rate at which energy is released in the body.

Phosphates are also a component of phospholipids, which promote the emulsification and transport of fats and fatty acids as well as the permeability of cell membranes.

Phosphorus is an essential constituent of nucleic acids and nucleoproteins in cell nuclei, which play a key role in reproduction, transmission of hereditary traits, cell division, and protein synthesis within the cells. In other words, phosphorus is needed to combine with protein to form cells.

Phosphorus seems to play an important part in the activity of certain vitamins of the B group. It also is involved in the output of nervous energy.

Deficiency: A phosphorus deficiency seldom, if ever, develops in most people because of its wide distribution in food. But persons not knowledgeable about nutrition and consuming typical vegetarian-type diets (especially those low in milk products) may encounter a lack of phosphorus in their diet. The young athlete may encounter a deficiency of this mineral if his rapidly growing muscles use the phosphorus from food and deprive the bones of it. A lack of phosphorus also results in poor teeth that are more subject to decay in later life.

Deficiencies also are seen in persons receiving antacids over long periods and in certain stress situations such as bone fractures. Such persons often show weakness, bone pain, demineralization of bone, and loss of calcium.

Sources: Most plant and animal foods contain appreciable amounts of phosphorus. Almost every good source of calcium provides phosphorus, and a diet that supplies adequate amounts of protein usually is adequate for phosphorus. The best sources of this mineral are the organ meats, liver, heart, and kidney. Beef, pork, veal, fowl, fish, milk, and cheese are also high in phosphorus. Other good sources are soybeans and other dried beans, peas, eggs, and whole-grain cereals. The calcium-poor foods (meats and cereal) are phosphorus-rich.

Edible roots, stems, and flowerets of plants contain calcium *and* phosphorus. Plants concentrate calcium in the green leaves (dark green leaves of all kinds) and phosphorus in the seeds (grains).

A vegetarian who disdains products such as eggs, milk, and seafood has a nip-and-tuck tangle with the calcium-phosphorus-vitamin D triad unless he informs himself well and carefully.

Recommended Allowance: The allowance for a normal adult is 800 mg a day. A rather wide variation of the calcium:phosphorus ratio in the diet can be tolerated provided the supply of vitamin D is adequate.

MAGNESIUM

Magnesium is a silvery-white metal similar in function to calcium and phosphorus. Magnesium, a major mineral component of seawater from which life and chlorophyll originally evolved, is the central component of chlorophyll. It is absolutely essential in plants for making glucose and oxygen from sunlight, water, and carbon dioxide.

The human body contains about 20 to 28 grams of magnesium, over half of which is found in the complex salts that make up bone. The remainder is found chiefly in the cells of soft tissues, especially the liver and skeletal muscles. A large fraction of the remainder is found within cells, and a very small amount is present in the fluids surrounding them. The body can store magnesium in the bones.

Function: The primary function of magnesium appears to be as an activator of certain enzymes in the body, particularly those related to carbohydrate metabolism (reactions that synthesize glucose to glycogen in the liver and muscles). This is of particular importance to athletes.

Magnesium is necessary for regulation of body temperature, and it also takes part in the regulation of the acid-base balance of the body. Furthermore, it is essential for synthesis of protein.

Small amounts of magnesium are present in the body fluids and take part in the transfer by osmosis of water into and out of the cells. Magnesium is important in maintaining normal muscle function, and in the conduction of nerve impulses.

Magnesium is a component of an especially valuable electrolyte in the body fluid for distance runners. Magnesium has been isolated as one of two important minerals lost during athletic competition, especially in hot weather. (Potassium is the other.)

Deficiency: Deficiences are rare—especially if the diet contains a reasonable amount of green vegetables. Magnesium deficiencies do not occur in normal persons who eat a variety of traditional wholesome foods. Deficiency symptoms are slow to develop in humans because of reserve stores in the body. The normal kidney is able to conserve magnesium in borderline intakes, thus preventing greater deficiencies from occurring.

Behavioral disturbances, delirium, and depression are seen as well as weakness, tremors, vertigo, tetany, spasms, convulsions, and other problems similar to those seen clinically in calcium deficiency. Similar nervous and muscular excitability is seen in magnesium deficiency.

One of the symptoms of magnesium deficiency is muscle cramping; therefore, an endurance athlete should be concerned with consuming foods and liquids containing magnesium rather than gobbling salt tablets or drinking commercial salt-replacement solutions.

Sources: Good sources of magnesium are whole grains, nuts, beans, and green leafy vegetables. Animal products—including meat and milk—are only poor to fair sources. Processing of foods can result in high losses. Distribution of magnesium in foods tends to follow that of phosphorus and some proteins!

Recommended Allowance: The magnesium requirement depends upon body size and composition of the diet. High calcium in the diet is known to compete with the absorption of magnesium. Protein, phosphorus, and vitamin D levels also influence the requirement. The allowances are roughly 50 percent higher than minimal requirements (which range between 200 and 300 mg per day for adults) to allow for individual differences, normal stresses, and variations in diet composition.

Average allowances are:

400 mg—active athletes
350 mg—males
300 mg—females

Animal protein-rich diets and alcohol consumption might hinder the absorption of magnesium from the intestine and correspondingly raise the magnesium requirements.

Magnesium salts (like those of calcium) are usually rather insoluble, so their absorption is rather low and occurs in the small intestine. Normally, about one-third of ingested magnesium is absorbed.

TABLE 6-1   FOODS CONTAINING MAGNESIUM*

Food Source	Amount	Milligrams of Magnesium
Nuts and Seeds		
Peanuts	¼ cup	76
Peanut butter	2 tablespoons	56
Cashews	5 nuts	28
Sesame seeds	1 tablespoon	17
Filberts	5 nuts	14
Sunflower seeds	¼ cup	14
Grains and Grain Products		
Whole wheat flour	½ cup	68
Wheat germ	2 tablespoons	35
Wheat bran	2 tablespoons	32
Rice, brown (cooked)	½ cup	29
Oatmeal (cooked)	½ cup	25
Bread, whole wheat	1 slice	22
Macaroni (cooked)	½ cup	13
Bread, white	1 slice	6

Food Source	Amount	Milligrams of Magnesium
Legumes		
Soybeans, dry	¼ cup	139
Soybean flour, full fat	½ cup	87
Lentils, dry	¼ cup	38
Vegetables		
Beet greens	4 ounces	120
Spinach	4 ounces	100
Brussel sprouts	5 large	74
Potato, white, unpeeled	1 medium	51
Potato, sweet	1 medium	50
Broccoli stalks	2 medium	48
Beets	3 medium	40
Parsnips	1 medium	40
Fruits		
Banana	1 medium	39
Grapefruit	½ medium	17
Orange	1 medium	14
Orange juice	½ cup	14
Apple	1 medium	13
Miscellaneous		
Chocolate, sweet	1 ounce	30
Cocoa, dry	1 tablespoon	21
Yeast, brewer's	1 tablespoon	18

* Figures are adapted from U.S. Department of Agriculture Handbook No. 8, *Composition of Foods — Raw, Processed, Prepared*, approved for reprinting October, 1975.

POTASSIUM

Potassium, named in 1807 from the word "potash," the alkaline ash of vegetable substances, is one of the most abundant elements. Potassium belongs to the same family of elements as sodium, and it unites with chlorine to form potassium chloride—also a salt. It can also combine with other elements to form other potassium salts.

Potassium is one of the many minerals of particular interest and concern to athletes. Potassium is a component of one of the electrolytes present in body fluids.

The need for potassium is increased when there is growth or development of lean tissue since potassium is an essential ingredient for muscle growth. Because potassium is a nearly constant component of lean body tissue, one method of estimating the amount of lean tissue is by measuring the amount of potassium present. This is done by counting the amount of radioactive potassium present, which is always in a constant ratio to ordinary potassium.

Potassium has been isolated as one of two important minerals lost during athletic competition, especially in hot weather. Magnesium is the other mineral.

Function: Potassium is involved primarily with cellular enzyme function. Potassium (and sodium) are components in the main body electrolytes. The major function of electrolytes is to control and maintain the correct rate of fluid exchange within various fluid compartments of the body. Potassium (and sodium) salts are the main preservers of our bodily inner sea.

Potassium phosphate salts are a vital part of the basic metabolic machinery inside the cells. Cells cannot function properly without adequate amounts of potassium salts. Most of the body's sodium is located in extracellular fluids, whereas most of the potassium is within the cells; thus, osmosis is made possible, and a normal water balance is maintained. In this way the constant flow of dissolved nutrients into the cell and waste products out of the cell is properly regulated.

The proper maintenance of both fluid and electrolyte balance is also of critical importance, especially during exercise in warm environments. It is common for athletes, and others, who sweat profusely during work to increase their normal salt and fluid intake automatically, independent of thirst, to offset the effects of dehydration. The crucial need is to replace water lost through sweating.

Other important functions of the electrolytes include maintaining the proper electrical gradients around the nerve membranes for the transmission of nerve impulses. Too much potassium affects the cells that control the heartbeat. This may cause the heart to slow or even stop. Surgeons use potassium to stop the heart when doing open heart surgery.

The kidneys normally eliminate excess potassium that the body does not need.

Deficiency: Potassium is important inside the cells making up the muscle fibers of the heart since a low level can lead to irregularities of the heart. Deficiency of potassium results in muscular weakness or paralysis.

When sweating excessively, the body loses the electrolytes present in sweat. These conditions impair heat tolerance and exercise performance. If electrolytes, especially water, are not replaced, severe dysfunction in the form of heat cramps and heat stroke can occur.

In most cases, deficiency results from a combination of poor diet and excessive loss of potassium due to severe diarrhea.

A low potassium level is more common now because of new medicines used to eliminate body water, the so-called water pills; they cause the kidneys to flush out sodium and also potassium. These medicines are commonly used for people who have fluid retention. As a result, the more water pills prescribed, the greater the need to emphasize the importance of a diet that provides an adequate amount of potassium.

Potassium is also an energy mineral. Without it you may feel lackadaisical.

Sources: The ordinary diet usually contains enough potassium, if carbohydrate and protein intake are adequate, because potassium is widely distributed in foods of both plant and animal origin.

The best food sources for potassium are fruits, such as bananas, cantaloupe, apricots, dates, and citrus fruits; lean meats, including chicken and liver; skim milk; dark green leafy vegetables; tomatoes; and raw carrots. Also, there are small amounts of potassium in all cereals.

Recommended Allowance: Adults need about 2.5 gm per day of potassium. It is wise to maintain a one-to-one ratio of sodium to potassium in the diet. Lower your salt intake and increase your potassium intake. Athletes take note!

SODIUM

Sodium, from the word "soda," is a very soft, white, silvery metal that burns on exposure to air, is widely distributed throughout nature, and is in abundant supply in all foods.

Sodium serves as a component of electrolyte; it is present in the body as electrically charged particles called ions. When an element such as sodium combines with another element such as chlorine, it forms a salt—in this case, sodium chloride, or ordinary table salt. Sodium and chlorine in salt are essential nutrients. Salt is approximately 40 percent sodium and 60 percent chlorine. Ordinary table salt ($NaCl$) and baking soda ($NaHCO_3$) are common and familiar forms of the element.

Sodium is found primarily in body fluids in the spaces between cells (the extracellular fluids). Athletes will be interested to know that it is the chief metallic ion in body sweat; a significant amount can be lost in profuse and protracted sweating.

Function: Although sodium and chlorine are the two elements that combine to form sodium chloride, each has separate functions in the body. Sodium is involved primarily with the maintenance of osmotic equilibrium and body fluid volume, and it is found mainly in blood plasma and in fluids outside the body cells, where it helps to maintain normal water balance inside and outside the cells. Potassium and sodium determine the amount of water held in the tissues. Sodium is a key element in regulation of body water and acid-base balance.

Deficiency: A water-salt imbalance and draining of the body's electrolyte reserve lead to all sorts of complications. Long runs in hot weather require special attention to drinking habits and the kinds of liquids one drinks.

Salt tablets usually are not necessary. (A salt tablet is like a piece of brine, and when it rests in the stomach, it can cause nausea and vomiting.) If you anticipate perspiring, take a little extra salt with your food beforehand. During an athletic contest, take a little salt with water or salt a piece of fruit. You might have a cup of bouillon after the contest. But don't overdo it. The body can't store salt, and you might induce the cramps and muscular weakness you were trying to avoid.

Sources: This mineral is abundantly present in the average American diet because of the sodium in the salt added to food. Other sources of added sodium are monosodium glutamate (MSG), soy sauce, and baking powder. Water supplies are quite variable in sodium content but can add significantly to the daily total intake. Sodium-rich foods come from animal sources such as meat, fish, poultry, eggs, and milk. Good sources of sodium are cheese, milk, and shellfish. Cereals, fruits, and vegetables are low in this nutrient unless it is added in processing. Many processed foods, such as ham, bacon, bread, and crackers, have a high sodium content because salt or sodium compounds are added in processing.

Recommended Allowance: Sodium and potassium are so abundant in the average diet that the problem tends to be one of excess (at least of sodium). The body has such effective means of conserving sodium when it is scarce—by gradually decreasing the salt concentration of sweat—and of ridding the body of any excess via the urine that it is difficult to establish a minimum daily requirement for this nutrient.

The average daily American intake is 10 to 15 gm of salt, or about 5 gm of sodium. A safe lower intake level is thought to be about 2.5 gm of sodium per day. If sweating loss is high, there might be need for additional salt in the diet, but the usual intake, 10 to 15 gm of salt, is more than sufficient to cover the loss that occurs with most physical work or moderate heat exposure. Sweat contains up to 1 gm of sodium per liter, so the usual sodium intake (5 gm per day) allows for at least 4 liters of sweat after all other sodium needs are met.

For persons who participate in a heavy workout in a hot climate under hot conditions, salt intake should be increased to about 7 gm per day. This is best accomplished by salting food or by adding salt to drinking water used to replace the water lost as sweat.

Sweat is hypotonic, that is, it contains a lower concentration of salt than the physiological saline level (0.9 percent).

Thus, fluid drunk for replacement also must be less concentrated than the extracellular fluid. A good solution should have 2 gm of salt per liter (2 scant teaspoons of salt per gallon). On a warm day a simple safeguard (for salt requirement) is to drink a cup of bouillon several hours prior to the athletic event.

SULFUR

Sulfur is a solid, non-metallic element found in great quantities in nature. It is necessary for the growth of plants and animals, and it is found in many vegetables such as onions, cabbage, and horseradish. It also is present in eggs, where a sulfur compound makes the strong odor noticeable when the eggs become spoiled.

Sulfur is present in all body tissues and is essential to life. The body can build amino acids from sugars, starches, and fats if the few necessary sulfurs are included in the diet. Sulfur is a part of two vitamins, thiamine and biotin. The complete function of sulfur has not yet been established.

IRON

The total amount of iron in the human body is approximately 5 grams (about one-sixth of an ounce). Iron is stored in combination with proteins in the liver, spleen, and bone marrow, normally constituting about 25 to 30 percent of the iron in the whole body. About 5 percent of the iron is found in other tissues of the body, and the largest portion of iron, about 65 percent, is present in the blood in molecules of hemoglobin, which gives blood its color and increases its oxygen-carrying capacity about 65 times.

Iron was found to be a treatment for anemia in the seventeenth century; it was a major ingredient of old-time patent medicines. It is unfortunate that even though the need for iron was discovered long ago and it is the cheapest and most common of all metals, iron deficiency is the most widespread nutrient deficiency in the United States today.

All endurance athletes should be concerned with building up and maintaining a high proportion of hemoglobin in their blood.

Function: Much of the iron in our bodies combines with protein to make hemoglobin, the red substance in the blood that carries oxygen to the cells. The amount of oxygen the blood can carry to muscle tissues is dependent on the amount of hemoglobin in the blood.

The hemoglobin in each red blood cell picks up oxygen from the lungs and carries it throughout the body, supplying it to each cell for its energy processes. The body needs oxygen to burn the carbohydrates, fats, and proteins and so release their energy. When oxygenated, the blood is red. When the hemoglobin has given up its oxygen to a cell, it turns a bluish color. Thus, arterial blood leaving the heart is red. Venous blood returning to the heart is bluish.

Deficiency: Women tend to be more deficient in iron than men. Deficiencies often occur in females who have heavy menstrual periods.

Due to lack of iron, the level of hemoglobin in the red cells is reduced, and the red cells themselves are smaller. Iron deficiency reduces the oxygen-carrying capacity of the blood, resulting in such symptoms as lack of energy and vitality, lack of appetite, paleness of skin, weakness, fatigue and sleepiness, becoming easily winded, and even emotional depression.

Sources: The iron in animal food is generally believed to be in more available form than that in vegetable foods. Liver is the richest iron source. Other sources are red meats (especially organ meats), eggs, whole grains, molasses, dark green leafy vegetables, dried prunes, raisins, and apricots.

Foods supplying iron but only in small amounts are whole grain and enriched bread and cereals.

Recommended Allowance: Males 12-18 years old need 18 mg of iron; over 18, 10 mg. Females 10-55 years old need 18 mg; over 55, 10 mg. Children up to 3 years old need 15 mg; those 3-10 years old require 10 mg.

The need for iron varies at different ages and under different conditions. The demand is especially high during infancy, adolescence, and pregnancy. Children require varying amounts according to their size.

Since only about one-tenth of the iron in food is absorbed into the body, it is important that a good supply of foods rich in iron be included in the diet each day. However, the body is able to recycle iron and carefully reuses any that is broken down by the cells. Only the small amounts of iron lost in the urine, sweat, hair, sloughed off skin, nails, and by menstruation need to be replaced.

Iron is present in many of our favorite foods, yet iron shortages are among the chief concerns of today's food scientists. Valuable iron is lost because of refining and processing our food supply. Increased food enrichment with iron is one partial solution.

So-called progress also might be a reason for decreased iron in our diet; cast iron cooking equipment no longer receives the use that it did in grandmother's time.

TABLE 6-2   FOODS CONTAINING IRON*

Food Source	Amount	Milligrams of Iron
Meats		
Liver, lamb	3 ounces	13.4
Liver, beef	4 ounces	10.0
Hamburger, lean	4 ounces	3.6
Ham	4 ounces	3.2
Most meats	4 ounces	3.0-4.0
Chicken breast	1/2 breast	1.3
Sea Foods		
Oysters, shrimps	3 ounces	2.5-5.5
Tuna (canned in oil)	3 ounces	1.6
Legumes		
Beans, lima (cooked)	1/2 cup	3.0
Soybeans (cooked)	1/2 cup	2.5
Peas, split (cooked)	1/2 cup	2.1

Food Source	Amount	Milligrams of Iron
Vegetables		
Green, leafy (cooked)	½ cup	0.8-2.0
Other vegetables	½ cup	0.7-2.1
Fruits (dried)		
Figs	4 small	1.8
Apricots	4 halves	1.7
Prunes	4-5 medium	1.2
Raisins	2 tablespoons	0.7
Dates, pitted	2 tablespoons	0.6
Fruits, fresh		
Watermelon	1 wedge (4x8")	2.1
Italian plums	½ cup	1.1
Banana	1 medium	0.8
Most fruits	½ cup	0.3-0.8
Nuts		
Most nuts	¼ cup	1.2-1.8
Bread and Cereals		
Bran flakes, 40%	1 cup	12.3
Rice, enriched-cooked	½ cup	0.9
Bread, whole wheat	1 slice	0.8
Oatmeal (cooked)	½ cup	0.7
Macaroni (cooked)	½ cup	0.7
Cereals: oats, corn, wheat, rice (dry) (unenriched)	1 cup	0.2-0.7
(enriched-read label for enrichment)		up to 10.0
Miscellaneous		
Prune juice	½ cup	5.3
Molasses, blackstrap	1 tablespoon	3.2
Beans, baked with pork and molasses	½ cup	3.0
Egg, whole	1 large	1.1
Molasses, light	1 tablespoon	0.9
Milk, skim	1 cup	0.1

*Adapted from "Nutritive Value of Foods," Home and Garden Bulletin No. 72, United States Department of Agriculture, revised January, 1971.

IODINE

Iodine is one of the chemical elements closely related to fluorine, bromine, and chlorine.

Iodine is found widely distributed in small amounts in various minerals, usually combined with sodium and potassium. Estimates of the total amount in the body range from 15 to 30 mg (about the size of a match head), and of this small amount about three-fifths is concentrated in the thyroid gland (the rest is mostly in the circulating blood). Iodine is absorbed from the alimentary tract; approximately 30 percent is removed by the thyroid gland, where it is stored.

Function: In the thyroid gland, iodine becomes part of the hormone that influences the rate of energy metabolism in cells. Iodine is one of the most important elements necessary for growth and the maintenance of life. Almost all living things require iodine.

Deficiency: Iodine deficiency shows up as goiter, an enlargement of the thyroid gland in the neck.

If the deficiency continues, this gland continues to enlarge in an attempt to compensate for the shortage of iodine, which is essential for the production of its hormones.

Sources: Some areas of the United States called the "Goiter Belt" have soil that is deficient in iodine. The iodine content of food depends upon the soil in which it grows. Vegetables grown in soil containing iodine have this mineral; those grown in soil deficient in iodine have little or none.

In 1924 the goiter problem was solved by adding a little iodine to table salt. The iodization of salt is not mandatory, but under a 1972 U.S. Food and Drug Administration regulation, non-iodized salt must carry the statement: "This salt does not supply iodine, a necessary nutrient."

Unfortunately, the old iodine-goiter problem is so nearly forgotten that the use of iodized salt has been declining—a source of concern to doctors and nutritionists. There is absolutely no harm possible from the amount of iodine added to table salt. The American Medical Association urges that Americans use *only* iodized salt because of the goiter risk in using salt that has *not* been iodized.

Foods from the sea are the richest natural sources of iodine. Small amounts of iodine can be added to the water supply as an aid in preventing goiter.

Recommended Allowance: Between 100 and 150 micrograms. Only 50 to 75 micrograms of iodine are needed to prevent goiter. That tiny amount is essential to the normal function of the important thyroid gland and the production of key thyroid hormones.

ZINC

Zinc, a bluish-white metal, is an essential trace element. A total of about 2 grams is present in an adult human body, which is thought to be about a 200-day supply for nutritional needs. In the blood, three-fourths of the zinc is in the red cells.

Function: In man, zinc is essential for general growth of all tissues (including stature); it is also necessary for wound healing, prevention of anemia, and the normal growth of genital organs. Zinc activates enzymes that function in the digestion of proteins. Zinc assists a reaction that is important in the transport of carbon dioxide via the red blood cells from the tissues to the lungs, where it can be exhaled. Zinc is a constituent of the hormone insulin, secreted by the pancreas and important in carbohydrate metabolism.

Deficiency: Deficiencies are rarely seen in the United States. They include delayed wound-healing and loss of the sense of taste.

Sources: Zinc occurs widely in plant and animal tissues. It is present in all natural foods, but it is low in fruits and vegetables and it is especially low in refined foods. Whole-grain cereals are rich in zinc, but because of the presence of other substances, such as phytin, the zinc may not be completely available for absorption.

Oysters are an especially rich source of zinc, as are red meat, fish, egg yolks, and milk.

Recommended Allowance: The average American diet supplies about 10 to 15 mg of zinc per day, and about half of this amount is absorbed by the body. That quantity has been found to be sufficient to prevent deficiencies.

There is no "recommended allowance," but about 6 mg has been suggested as a tentative requirement for children.

CHLORINE

Chlorine is an essential element for all higher animals, including man. Chlorine is a very toxic yellow-green gas in its elemental form. In nature it always exists combined with another element. A common form is sodium chloride (NaCl); to us, common table salt. It is also used as a water purifier and bleach.

Function: Chlorine is one of three minerals in the body that serve as components of electrolytes; the other two minerals are sodium and potassium. All three are present in the body in relatively large amounts and are required in the diet in larger quantities than the "trace elements." Electrolytes are water solutions of salts, acids, and alkalies.

The chloride electrolyte is involved in the important acid-base maintenance of the body. In addition, chlorine has a special function in forming hydrochloric acid (HCl). Chlorine reacts with hydrogen and dissolves readily in water, making hydrochloric acid, which is present in gastric juice as an aid to the digestion of food in the stomach. Hydrochloric acid is necessary for proper absorption of vitamin B-12 and iron, and it suppresses growth of microorganisms that enter the stomach with our food and liquids.

Deficiency: Loss of chloride generally parallels that of sodium; a separate deficiency occurs only when there is loss of chloride due to vomiting.

Sources: The most common source of chlorine is (along with sodium) common table salt, but if sodium is restricted because of heart, liver or kidney problems, a chloride-containing salt substitute is available.

Recommended Allowance: The usual diet provides more than enough of this mineral.

FLUORINE

Fluorine is an essential nutrient for man; it is a very reactive gas, present in soil, water, and in small amounts in almost all plant and animal foods (as a fluoride). Like many other trace elements, in too large amounts it can have toxic effects.

Fluorine is readily absorbed from the intestine and is distributed widely in the body, with highest concentrations in the teeth and bones.

Function: Fluorine is necessary for maximum resistance to dental decay.

A long-term intake of fluoride (at one part per million, the same as for preventing tooth decay) will delay, or perhaps prevent, one manifestation of aging—osteoporosis. Osteoporosis is a gradual leaching out of minerals—particularly calcium, as well as protein—from the bones, leaving them brittle, porous, and easy to break. The body needs vitamin D and fluorine for proper metabolism of both calcium and protein.

Apparently, fluoride is necessary to "fix," or hold, calcium salts in the bones, particularly during hormonal changes and when the ability to absorb calcium from the intestine decreases, which comes with aging. So far, evidence indicates that a high fluoride intake must begin many years before it is apparently necessary, just as other dietary changes must take place long before middle age if we are to prevent degenerative diseases.

Deficiency: Many areas of the U.S. have soils and water supplies low in fluorine and calcium, resulting in poor bone and teeth formations and dental decay.

Sources: Regulation of the fluorine content of water by addition of fluorides in localities where there is a deficiency, to a range of 0.7 to 1.2 parts per million for prevention of tooth decay, is now a scientifically accepted, safe, economical, and efficient public health measure for supplying this element.

Seafood, such as fish eaten with bones (salmon, sardines, etc.), and tea (about 0.2 to 0.3 mg per cup) are among the highest sources. Bone meal is also very rich in fluorine; some people use it as a mineral supplement. But the most reliable sources of fluorine are fluoridated water and fluoridated salt.

Fluorine tablets and fluorine toothpastes also are available and reliable sources of this nutrient but are more expensive than fluoridated water or salt.

Recommended Allowance: A normal day's diet in the U.S. contains about 0.3 to 0.6 mg of fluorine (as fluorides), not including the amount in drinking water. Including drinking water, normal intake would be 1 to 2.5 mg per day.

Excess of fluorine is indicated by a mottling of tooth enamel. Excess fluorine is excreted in the urine.

COPPER

Copper was discovered in prehistoric times, but not until about 50 years ago was its importance in nutrition realized. A total of approximately 75 to 150 mg of copper is present in the human adult body.

Function: Copper, in trace amounts, helps the body to use iron in building red blood cells; it also assists in the metabolism of glucose and release of energy, the formation of phospholipids in the nerve walls, and the formation of connective tissue.

Deficiency: An insufficient amount of iron and copper in the diet results in a reduction of hemoglobin, which, in turn, reduces the power of the blood to carry oxygen. The result is a condition known as nutritional anemia. This disease is characterized by paleness of skin and membranes. Listlessness, often mistaken for laziness, is noted, especially in children. Weakness also is evident when iron and copper are lacking.

Sources: Copper occurs along with other mineral elements in most natural foods. Richest sources are organ meats, oysters, fish, meat, dried legumes, whole-grain cereals, nuts, potatoes, and cocoa. The amount of copper in the diet depends both on the choice of foods and the locality in which they are produced. Some soils are more copper-rich than others.

Copper cooking utensils contribute to the copper needed in the diet. Copper rollers used in food processing also contribute to the copper content of food.

Recommended Allowance: Only minute amounts are needed. Deficiency is unlikely with a varied diet.

The requirement for copper seems to be about 2 milligrams daily. The average American gets that much and quite a bit more from his food.

Of the usual day's intake of copper (2 to 5 mg), about 30 percent is absorbed in the upper small intestine or stomach. Excess copper is excreted normally through the bile.

CHROMIUM

Acting in cooperation with insulin, chromium is required for glucose utilization. A deficiency can produce a diabetes-like condition. Good sources are dried brewer's yeast, whole-grain cereals, and liver.

SELENIUM

Selenium appears to have a "sparing action" on vitamin E, which means that it can serve as a partial substitute. A variety of problems occur in animals deficient in selenium and vitamin E, and from the important experiments that have been done on animals, it seems certain that selenium is important to man.

The selenium content of foods depends on the amount available to the growing plant or animal. Selenium protects against the active and chronic toxic effects of cadmium and mercury. Thus, a given concentration of cadmium or mercury in the environment can be toxic or harmless depending on the concentration of selenium present. Selenium is one of the most toxic elements in the environment of earth.

MANGANESE

Manganese is needed for normal tendon and bone structure

and is part of some enzymes. Manganese is abundant in many foods, especially bran, coffee, tea, nuts, peas, and beans. A deficiency in humans is unknown.

COBALT

Cobalt by itself is not essential in the body, but it is a part of vitamin B-12, which is a necessary nutrient.

Vegetarians who do not eat any meat, eggs, or dairy products can become vitamin B-12 deficient because it occurs only in trace amounts in plant products. No animal can manufacture vitamin B-12 in its tissues (only in the intestine). To a very limited extent, vitamin B-12 can be synthesized by microorganisms working on cobalt in humans. This probably explains why true vegetarians can live many years without vitamin B-12 itself in the diet.

Synthesis in the intestine is not certain at all in man, so we generally regard man's need of cobalt in terms of the intact vitamin B-12 molecule and not in terms of inorganic cobalt itself.

Cobalt ions are distributed throughout the body, especially in the liver and heart, and they do not accumulate with age. Cobalt is present in almost all foods in varying amounts; but our real concern is with vitamin B-12 rather than cobalt.

A normal day's intake of 150 to 600 mg of inorganic cobalt is far greater than any possible requirement.

NICKEL

Nickel is included among the essential trace elements because of reports of its presence in a serum protein in rabbits and man (called nickeloplasmin) and its apparent requirement by chickens.

Nickel is present in high levels in ribonucleic acids. It is widely distributed in foods, especially in plant foods. A deficiency in man never has been seen and would be unlikely to occur except under unusual conditions. A normal diet supplies about 0.3 mg to 0.6 mg per day; requirement for the element would be less than this. Nickel is only mildly toxic in animals.

TIN

Tin is widely distributed in foods of animal and plant origin, and a deficiency in man or animals under normal conditions would not be expected to occur.

The most common use of tin is in the "tin can," in which a thin inner coat of tin lines a steel can. Tin is only mildly toxic, and if acid fruit juices or similar products dissolve appreciable amounts of tin from a tin-plated can, the metal is not well-absorbed by man (though the iron might be). High levels of tin have been found in canned pineapple and citrus juices, but such amounts do not appear to be toxic. (Generally, cans containing acid juices now are lacquered.)

A normal tin intake is probably in the range of 1.5 to 5 mg a day, depending on the amount of canned food eaten. The requirement for man is not known but would be expected to be slightly less than 1 mg a day. Tin has been found to have a growth-promoting effect on rats.

MOLYBDENUM

Molybdenum is a component of the essential enzyme xanthine dehydrogenase and other enzymes. It is a factor in carbohydrate metabolism. The need for molybdenum is minute, and human deficiencies are not known.

Molybdenum is widely distributed in foods in very small amounts. Legumes, cereals, organ meats, and yeast are considered foods with most molybdenum present. It is well-utilized by the body and excess is excreted in the urine. A normal day's intake is about 0.1 to 0.4 mg. The human requirement is unknown.

SILICON

The element silicon (from the Latin word *silex*, meaning "flint") is the most abundant mineral element on earth. Its most common form is silicon dioxide (SiO_2), or sand, from which glass is made.

Silicon is needed in microgram amounts for normal growth and bone development. It constitutes a major nutrition discovery.

VANADIUM

Vanadium is known to be a catalyst in several biological systems and to be present in higher-than-normal concentrations in teeth.

No special deficiency signs have been noted other than poor growth. Vanadium requirements for man would be about 0.1 to 0.3 mg per day. Normal diets contain about ten times that amount, so deficiencies are rare under usual conditions. The amount of vanadium in our food and in the environment appears to be considerably lower than the toxic level.

CADMIUM, LEAD, AND MERCURY

Cadmium has been found associated with zinc, as well as with lead and mercury. This element has been found to be harmful and has no demonstrated essential function. Cadmium interferes with the functions of such essential elements as iron, copper, and calcium.

People exposed to large amounts of cadmium might develop anemia, kidney damage, and, finally, marked bone mineral loss. These effects are reduced with adequate intake of zinc, iron, copper, calcium, manganese, and ascorbic acid—in other words, a normal diet.

Cadmium, lead, and mercury all are metallic elements present in toxic amounts in our environment. Mercury occurs naturally in small amounts, but because of increased concentration in industrial wastes, some of our seafood contains mercury at toxic levels.

Lead has been found in high concentrations in soils and plants near highways due to discharges from automobile engines. There is a danger that lead in paint can be ingested by children, and lead glazes on pottery react harmfully with food, especially citrus juices.

One cannot completely avoid eating traces of toxic elements no matter how careful one is, but be aware of the sources and try to use safeguards.

FOOD AND NUTRITION BOARD, NATIONAL ACADEMY OF SCIENCES—NATIONAL RESEARCH COUNCIL RECOMMENDED DAILY DIETARY ALLOWANCES,[1] revised 1974. (designed for the maintenance of good nutrition of practically all healthy people in the United States)

	Age (yr.)	Weight (kg.)	Weight (lb.)	Height (cm.)	Height (in.)	Energy (kcal)[2]	Protein (gm.)	Fat-Soluble Vitamins Vitamin A Activity (re)[3]	Vitamin A Activity (i.u.)	Vitamin D (i.u.)	Vitamin E Activity[5] (i.u.)
Infants	0.0 to 0.5	6	14	60	24	Kg. x 117	Kg. x 2.2	420[4]	1,400	400	4
	0.5 to 1.0	9	20	71	28	Kg. x 108	Kg. x 2.0	400	2,000	400	5
Children	1 to 3	13	28	86	34	1,300	23	400	2,000	400	7
	4 to 6	20	44	110	44	1,800	30	500	2,500	400	9
	7 to 10	30	66	135	54	2,400	36	700	3,300	400	10
Men	11 to 14	44	97	158	63	2,800	44	1,000	5,000	400	12
	15 to 18	61	134	172	69	3,000	54	1,000	5,000	400	15
	19 to 22	67	147	172	69	3,000	54	1,000	5,000	400	15
	23 to 50	70	154	172	69	2,700	56	1,000	5,000		15
	51+	70	154	172	69	2,400	56	1,000	5,000		15
Women	11 to 14	44	97	155	62	2,400	44	800	4,000	400	12
	15 to 18	54	119	162	65	2,100	48	800	4,000	400	12
	19 to 22	58	128	162	65	2,100	46	800	4,000	400	12
	23 to 50	58	128	162	65	2,000	46	800	4,000		12
	51+	58	128	162	65	1,800	46	800	4,000		12
Pregnant						+300	+30	1,000	5,000	400	15
Lactating						+500	+20	1,200	6,000	400	15

[1]The allowances are intended to provide for individual variations among most normal persons as they live in the United States under usual environmental stresses. Diets should be based on a variety of common foods to provide other nutrients for which human requirements have been less well defined.

[2]Kilojoules (KJ) = 4.2 x kcal.

[3]Retinol equivalents.

[4]Assumed to be all as retinol in milk during the first 6 months of life. All subsequent intakes are assumed to be one half as retinol and one half as beta-carotene when calculated from international units. As retinol equivalents, three fourths are as retinol and one fourth as beta-carotene.

	Water-Soluble Vitamins							Minerals					
	Ascorbic Acid (mg.)	Folacin[6] (mcg.)	Niacin[7] (mg.)	Riboflavin (mg.)	Thiamine (mg.)	Vitamin B$_6$ (mg.)	Vitamin B$_{12}$ (mcg.)	Calcium (mg.)	Phosphorus (mg.)	Iodine (mcg.)	Iron (mg.)	Magnesium (mg.)	Zinc (mg.)
Infants	35	50	5	0.4	0.3	0.3	0.3	360	240	35	10	60	3
	35	50	8	0.6	0.5	0.4	0.3	540	400	45	15	70	5
Children	40	100	9	0.8	0.7	0.6	1.0	800	800	60	15	150	10
	40	200	12	1.1	0.9	0.9	1.5	800	800	80	10	200	10
	40	300	16	1.2	1.2	1.2	2.0	800	800	110	10	250	10
Men	45	400	18	1.5	1.4	1.6	3.0	1,200	1,200	130	18	350	15
	45	400	20	1.8	1.5	2.0	3.0	1,200	1,200	150	18	400	15
	45	400	20	1.8	1.5	2.0	3.0	800	800	140	10	350	15
	45	400	18	1.6	1.4	2.0	3.0	800	800	130	10	350	15
	45	400	16	1.5	1.2	2.0	3.0	800	800	110	10	350	15
Women	45	400	16	1.3	1.2	1.6	3.0	1,200	1,200	115	18	300	15
	45	400	14	1.4	1.1	2.0	3.0	1,200	1,200	115	18	300	15
	45	400	14	1.4	1.1	2.0	3.0	800	800	100	18	300	15
	45	400	13	1.2	1.0	2.0	3.0	800	800	100	18	300	15
	45	400	12	1.1	1.0	2.0	3.0	800	800	80	10	300	15
Pregnant	60	800	+2	+0.3	+0.3	2.5	4.0	1,200	1,200	125	18+[8]	450	20
Lactating	80	600	+4	+0.5	+0.3	2.5	4.0	1,200	1,200	150	18	450	25

[5] Total vitamin E activity, estimated to be 80% as alpha-tocopherol and 20% other tocopherols.

[6] The folacin allowances refer to dietary sources as determined by Lactobacillus casei assay. Pure forms of folacin may be effective in doses less than one fourth of the RDA.

[7] Although allowances are expressed as niacin, it is recognized that on the average 1 mg. of niacin is derived from each 60 mg. of dietary tryptophan.

[8] This increased requirement cannot be met by ordinary diets; therefore the use of supplemental iron is recommended.

7
Digestive Processes—
Putting It Together

Digestion is the process by which food is broken down into smaller particles so it can be of use to the body.

Digestion takes place along the alimentary canal. The mouth, esophagus, stomach, small intestine, and large intestine comprise the alimentary canal. It forms a continuous hollow tube with widenings in certain sections, such as the stomach and large intestine, that act as reservoirs where food is held for a period of time.

The alimentary tract has two main functions: 1) the muscular function of churning and physically breaking down food as well as moving the food through the alimentary canal, and 2) the secretory function of adding important digestive fluids that chemically break down the food in the tract.

Enzymes, which are a major constituent of digestive fluid, are vital in the chemical breakdown of food. There are hundreds of different enzymes; every internal organ has a unique variety produced by its secreting cells. Enzymes are also very specific; each one acts only on a certain type of substance in food.

Digestion, by muscular action and the chemical action of enzymes, takes place all along the alimentary canal. The digestive process begins in the mouth, where food is chewed and mixed with saliva. Saliva contains enzymes and therefore exerts chemical action on the food while it moistens it for swallowing.

While the food is still in the mouth, saliva's enzyme, amylase, begins breaking down starches into simple sugars, which are more easily absorbed. After food is swallowed, it passes through the esophagus by muscular action and into the stomach. The muscular contraction of the stomach mixes the food with gastric juice. Hydrochloric acid contained in this digestive juice breaks down food, activates enzymes, and coagulates proteins. Digestion of protein foods such as milk, eggs, and meat begins with the gastric juice in the stomach.

Chyme is food that has been thoroughly churned, partly digested, and changed to a thick liquid. In this thick state it passes from the stomach into the small intestine. Carbohydrate-rich foods tend to pass out of the stomach most quickly, then protein, fat next, and finally mixtures of protein and fat. The average time needed for the stomach to discharge an ordinary meal is about three hours. (The inclusion of some fat or fat and protein in a meal is useful to prevent hunger contractions before the next mealtime.)

The largest part of digestion and absorption takes place in the small intestine, which is about twenty feet in length. Several digestive juices act on the partly digested foods in the small intestine. Since the partially digested food is acidic due to the gastric juice, fluids from the liver and pancreas flow into the small intestine to neutralize the acid so that digestion can continue. Pancreatic juice, produced by the pancreas, contains enzymes that act on the partially digested protein. All protein-splitting enzymes are called proteases.

The liver, a small organ weighing about four pounds, produces bile that helps to emulsify and digest fats. The fat-splitting enzymes are lipases. They divide fats into fatty acids and glycerin. The juice containing this powerful enzyme is secreted into the small intestine. The liver is the body's chief chemical factory and warehouse. It is able to extract nutrients from the blood, store them, and release them into the bloodstream as needed. The liver also neutralizes toxic substances.

Completely digested food looks milky, is slightly acidic, and is thinner than chyme. Only when food particles are small enough to pass through the walls of the intestine and blood vessels are they completely digested. They are then absorbed by the tiny blood vessels and lymph vessels in the walls of the small intestine and carried into circulation. Food materials are then usable by the tissues, either as energy or for tissue building.

The large intestine is about twice the diameter of the small intestine but much shorter. This intestine is less muscularly active, and its function is to store waste food products and absorb small amounts of water and minerals. The waste materials that accumulate in the large intestine are roughage that cannot be digested in the body.

Food residues and excretory material often remain in the large intestine for 18 hours or more, and conditions for the growth of bacteria are more favorable here than in any other part of the alimentary canal. Some of these bacteria are beneficial, such as those that manufacture some vitamins.

About 48 hours after a meal, the last waste products are ready to leave the large intestine and be eliminated in the form of feces.

REFERENCES FOR FURTHER READING

Bogert, L.J., G.M. Briggs, and D.H. Calloway. *Nutrition and Physical Fitness.* 9th ed. Philadelphia: W.B. Saunders, 1973.

De Coursey, Dr. Russell. *The Human Organism.* 4th ed. New York: McGraw-Hill.

Lappe, F.M. *Diet for a Small Planet.* Rev. ed. New York: Ballantine Books, 1975.

Lincoln, A.F. *Nutrition Power for a More Powerful You.* Corvallis, Oregon: House of Lincoln, 1975.

National Academy of Sciences, National Research Council. *Recommended Dietary Allowances.* 8th ed. Washington, D.C.: National Academy of Sciences.

United States Department of Agriculture. "Nutritive Value of Foods," *Home and Garden Bulletin No. 72.* Washington, D.C.: U.S. Government Printing Office, 1971.

part 2

Nutritional Conditioning

8

From Nutrients to Energy, Growth, and Muscle

ENERGY FROM FOOD

We have learned that the sun is the prime source of all energy. But we get our body energy directly from plants and also indirectly from plants through animals. Only plants have the ability to grow by combining the energy from the sun with elements from the air and soil and water. The energy that is released in the body combines all the various materials from food, that came from plants and animals, to make the many different body tissues such as muscle, bone, and blood and to provide the energy for body processes that include breathing, digestion of food, and even the pumping of the heart. The process of releasing energy from food and using it in so many ways is one of the marvels of the body.

Calories—What Are They?

Energy is the ability to do work, and energy is released from food by oxidation, or burning. The energy that results from this process is expressed in terms of calories, which are units of heat. For the physicist, one calorie is the amount of energy (heat) required to raise the temperature of one gram of water one degree centigrade. The energy supplied in the food we eat and the energy we need for the work we do is measured in calories. But this latter calorie is a nutritionist calorie, which is 1,000 times larger: it is the amount of heat required to raise the temperature of one *kilogram* of water one degree centigrade. All further reference to calories in this book is to the nutritionist calorie sometimes referred to as a kcal.

ENERGY REQUIREMENTS FOR BASAL METABOLISM

In order to know how much food a person needs it is important to determine what is required for the internal working of one's body. Unlike a gasoline engine, our body can never be shut down. We go on breathing, our heart continues to pump, the liver and kidneys work constantly, and the brain's energy use is constant; in fact, the internal energy use scarcely varies whether we are sleeping or working.

Even though our body cannot be shut down, it can "idle." The time when the internal workings of the body can be at their lowest ebb, and the whole body be most completely at rest, is from 12 to 15 hours after the last meal. Lying quietly, relaxed but awake, in a comfortable environment, neither hot nor cold, are the conditions that allow for an accurate determination of minimum calorie needs. This "basal" energy expenditure goes on day in and day out throughout the entire 24 hours of the day; it is called "basal metabolism rate" (BMR).

Figuring Basal Metabolism Rate (BMR)

Basal metabolic energy needs are influenced by the secretions of the endocrine glands. These secretions are the primary regulators of the rate of metabolism of body cells.

Normal BMR is about one calorie burned per hour for each kilogram of body weight. To make it easier for most of us to calculate, a man can multiply his weight (stripped) in pounds by 11 to get his approximate BMR (150 x 11 = 1,650 calories per day). A woman's rate is about 10 percent less because, generally, men have more muscle and less fat than women. Since muscle burns more energy, more food can be consumed. A woman may multiply her weight in pounds by 11 and subtract 10 percent of that amount; or, for all practical purposes, she may just use the factor 10 instead of 11. This BMR formula is for the young adult. The BMR of a healthy adult man is about 1,600 to 1,800 calories per day; for women it is about 1,200 to 1,450 calories per day.

Adjusting BMR for Age

Basal metabolic energy requirements are influenced by age. The rate is higher in young people than in older individuals. It increases for some months after birth, and then it decreases (at first fairly rapidly, but later more gradually) up to and through adolescence. In adults there is a slow decline in basal rate with increasing age. A woman should subtract 5 calories for each year over 25 up to the age of 45; then subtract 15 calories more for each year over 45. For a woman of 40 this would mean cutting a total of 75 calories, or for a woman of 55 it would mean cutting a total of 250 calories from the daily BMR need.

A man at desired weight should take 10 calories off for each year over 25 years. Thus, a man of 60 could cut 350 calories from his earlier BMR need.

ENERGY REQUIREMENTS FOR EXTERNAL WORK AND MINOR NEEDS

The total allowance for energy requirement must cover amounts needed for *internal work* (basal metabolism) and *external work,* and also the *minor factors* of energy "cost" of the food intake, temperature of the environment, and especially growth allowance (discussed later).

It is difficult to figure energy needs for external work since one is usually not strenuously active throughout a day; everyone has periods of sitting, standing, arm movements, even times of deep concentration.

One realizes that every action takes energy. How many muscles, what size muscles, the rate of moving the muscles and how vigorously and for what length of time, are only a few of the variables that affect the estimating of the total calories needed for external work each day. Even a nutritionist admits that figuring energy needs is a big order.

Anyone wanting to figure caloric needs according to intensity of activity, may use these figures as a guide, i.e. add on to the BMR adjusted for age the following:

100 calories/hour for *sedentary activities:* includes watching television, reading, eating, studying and those activities done while sitting that require little arm movement.

150 calories/hour for *light activities:* includes dressing, undressing, shaving, washing, walking slowly, preparing food, and similar activities while standing; or rapid typing, or similar activities while sitting.

200 calories/hour for *moderate activity:* includes walking moderately fast, bicycling at moderate speed, golf, table tennis, and those activities done while standing that require moderate arm movement; activities done while sitting that require more vigorous arm movement.

300 calories/hour for *vigorous activity:* includes walking fast, jogging, down-hill skiing, gymnastic exercise, skating, dancing and horseback riding.

400 calories/hour for *strenuous activity:* includes running, swimming, sawing wood, walking uphill, cross-country skiing, tennis, horseback riding or other active sports.

Besides basal metabolism needs and the allowance for

external work (or physical activity), another important consideration in figuring energy requirement is the "cost" of the food intake. By "cost" is meant the amount of energy lost to the body's use because of the energy required in the digestive process. About 10 percent of the food intake is used in this way, which means that a 200 pound athlete consuming 4,000 calories, gets the benefit of only 3,600 of that amount.

Temperature also affects one's caloric needs; one needs more calories for heat energy in cold weather than in warm.

Periods of stress affects one's body needs—an emotionally tense person burns more calories than a relaxed one.

Athletic experience is also a factor in calculating caloric needs, since the experienced athlete has better coordination, greater skill, and more efficient movement—and therefore uses less energy.

ENERGY REQUIREMENTS FOR GROWTH

With growing children, it is important to provide energy over and above that required for the internal work of the body and for muscular activity in order that additional material may be available for increasing the body weight in growth. During rapid periods of growth, the increased allowance could be as much as 10 percent. As growth rate diminishes, the allowance needed per unit of body weight becomes smaller, even though the total food requirement is more because of the increased size.

In general, it is unwise to restrict caloric intake rigorously during the growing and developmental period of an athlete's life. There needs to be an extra allowance of food for the growth that occurs in adolescent years. On the other hand, the growing athlete who is overeating and overweight needs to restrict calories unless he or she is exercising hard to lose weight.

Good bone growth is important during this period, and an allowance should be provided for that, too. The team of calcium, phosphorous, proteins, and vitamins C and D builds bones. Milk and milk products provide most of the calcium for good bone growth. When bones are growing, their weakest parts are just above and below joints, such as the knee, ankle, elbow, or wrist, and near the ends of ribs. This is where the growing layer is forming new bone.

Many parents are overly concerned about their adolescent athlete not eating enough "to grow on." At this age there are considerable individual differences in development and growth patterns. Parents cannot do much about influencing the amount of growth. What they can do is provide regular mealtimes, varied foods, a well-balanced diet, and freedom for the athlete to choose the amount of food he wishes so that he will develop good eating habits without too much danger of becoming overweight. It is important at this age to guard against establishing patterns that might lead to a lifelong struggle with obesity.

Growth rates for high-school-age youth vary greatly but average about ten pounds per year, or approximately three or four pounds during the one-third of the year represented by an athletic season. In many states wrestlers are allowed a weight gain of one to two pounds during each of the winter months. That adequately allows for normal growth. Greater increases will, in most cases, represent unwanted additions of fat tissue.

The college competitor usually has achieved adult growth already. With proper control of caloric intake, he can expect to maintain a stable weight throughout the season. If he "bounces" in weight, he is not disciplining his eating habits.

The balance between the energy supplied and the energy needed is important to growth and weight. Consuming more calories than needed will result in undesirable weight gain; consuming not enough calories to meet needs will result in undesirable weight loss. In the teens one wants to gain enough weight for normal growth, but it is important to gain no more. Excess food goes into storage as an extra fat load! A daily weight check indicates whether or not calories consumed are sufficient. Weigh in at the same time each day, dressed in the same manner. Weight is the best guide as to whether you're eating too much or the wrong foods.

The following formula and chart may be used to estimate reasonable daily caloric requirements for moderate activity for youths. Additional calories would be needed for greater activity.

Age	10 years	11–14 years	15–18 years	19 years
Suggested calories per pound per day	33 calories	31 calories	26 calories	20 calories

Desirable weight × calories per pound = total calories needed per day.

ENERGY REQUIREMENTS FOR GAINING MUSCLE—NOT FAT

Gaining weight is easy for many athletes, especially if they enjoy eating. But gaining weight is not a prime advantage in most sports unless the added tissue can be developed for production of strength. Most athletes who want to increase weight are concerned about an increase in muscle tissue rather than fat.

The idea that a great deal of protein is necessary for muscular work still persists in spite of knowledge that energy for muscular activity comes primarily from carbohydrates and fats. The many "health foods" and protein, vitamin, and mineral supplements available on the market help to promote the idea that "lots of protein is necessary for muscle building."

Does protein build muscle? In one sense, yes, but you might be surprised to know that protein is second to water as a main constituent of body structures such as muscles, tendons, skin, and other tissues. If muscle tissue from our body were chemically analyzed, we would find that over 70 percent of it is composed of water, and only 22 percent of the muscle is protein.

A small amount of protein is necessary in the development

of muscle, but exercise, with concentrated effort in specific areas, is the important first step in muscle growth. Developing, firming, and strengthening muscles requires intense exercise. Exercise does not increase the need for protein, but exercise does increase the need for carbohydrates and fats, which are our most efficient sources of energy.

Providing large amounts of protein in excess of what one's body requires will do nothing to promote growth of muscle tissue. But if one is exercising, the chemical creatine within a growing muscle will be stimulated to react with myosin, a protein necessary for muscle growth.

Some protein is involved in muscle cell growth, but exercise must always precede and accompany that growth, and carbohydrates and fats are the most efficient sources of energy for that exercise. Thus, one needs some protein to develop muscles and keep them healthy, but developing, firming, and strengthening of muscle does not come *just from eating protein*.

A normal well-balanced diet will supply adequate amounts of protein to build muscles, but the proper exercise program must accompany the nutrition. Remember the carbohydrates and fats for energy, and include plenty of milk and green leafy vegetables for necessary vitamins and minerals. The minerals phosphorus, potassium, and magnesium are important to the development and strengthening of muscle tissue.

A person who is dieting and exercising with the goal of losing weight often is surprised to learn what really happens: through exercise, stored fat is used as energy; but the exercise develops muscle in the specific areas exercised, resulting in less weight loss than expected. Also, he may be surprised to discover that a lean, muscular person will weigh more than a fat, flabby person with a comparable body frame.

COMPOSITION OF MUSCLE AND FAT

Tissue	Water	Lipids (Fat)	Protein
Muscle	70%	7%	22%
Fat	22%	72%	6%

Protein Requirement

How much protein does one really need each day? Probably less than most Americans get. It is an almost universal belief among coaches, athletes, and the public that strenuous exercise increases protein requirement. The need for protein is *not* increased by physical activity but is controlled largely by body size.

The *suggested* amount of protein is about 1 gram for each kilogram (2.2 pounds) of body weight, which is about double the *minimum* needed for life. Allow a little more, or half again as much, if the athlete is still growing. We don't know the advantages—if any—of going above the minimum protein needed for life or the minimum for optimal growth. Actually, many athletes eat three to four times as much as is absolutely required and almost twice the recommended allowance, which already has a margin of safety.

High protein diets usually are based on meat and are high in saturated fats. Decreasing our consumption of animal protein and increasing our intake of vegetable protein to a ratio of about half and half would be healthier than consuming all animal protein. Since fish and poultry usually have less fat and also are slightly higher in protein than red meat, they are good protein choices.

For the average athlete the daily protein requirement usually can be met by including 3 average servings chosen from these animal foods: cheese, milk, meat, poultry, fish, and eggs. About 25 to 35 grams of protein can be obtained from this group. In a well-balanced diet one also eats legumes (such as beans and peas), peanuts or other nuts, cereal products (including breads), and vegetables, which will provide another 25 to 35 grams of protein. This can bring total protein consumption to 50 to 70 grams.

For those particularly concerned with figuring the cost of protein, the least expensive protein foods are dried legumes, cereal products, dark green leafy vegetables, and potatoes. Eggs and milk, particularly dried skim milk, usually are moderate in cost.

To figure the approximate individual recommended daily allowance of protein, divide body weight in pounds by 2 and multiply by 0.9 to get grams:

Example: $(132 \div 2) \times 0.9 = 66 \times 0.9 = 59.4$, or 60 grams.

Or divide body weight in pounds by 10 and multiply by 1/6 to get ounces:

Example: $(132 \div 10) \times 1/6 = 13.2 \times 1/6 = 2.2$ ounces. (1 oz. = 28 grams, so 2.2 oz. = 61.6 grams)

PROTEIN CONTENT
OF A VARIETY OF FOODS

Food	Per cent of Protein
Poultry	30
Fish	19-30
Pumpkin and other seeds	19-29
Lean meats	20-28
Wheat germ	26
Peanuts	26
Cheese, Cheddar	25
Cashews	24
Variety of nuts	10-17
Dry cereals	8-15
Eggs	13
Legumes	8-10
Breads	8-10
Milk	3-4
Cooked cereal oatmeal	2.0

9

From Nutrients to Fat and Weight Reduction

A WEIGHT (FAT) CONTROL PROGRAM FOR SCHOOLS

When more calories are ingested than are needed for growth requirements and energy expended, they are stored as fat.

Because most people in this country of plentiful food eat more than they need, "overweight" and "obese" are heard more frequently than "underweight" and "skinny." For evidence just observe an assembly of people or passersby on a street while waiting for someone. Overweight is common among young people also; consequently, a weight-control, or more correctly, a fat-control program is needed in a school athletic program.

Much misunderstanding arises because of a lack of knowledge of the physical requirements of a particular sport, the relationship of weight to these requirements, and the nutrition information to help in proper eating. Weight control programs can be invaluable to the success of the athlete and the coach and can be a factor in good cooperation between parents and school officials, also. Communication between coaches, athletes, and parents can lead to a more effective training program.

The following suggestions are offered for a weight- (fat-) control program for schools or organized groups:

1. Make instructional materials concerning the athletic program available to all athletes and their parents.
2. Set up a meeting, including parents, school officials, and the coaching staff for discussion of the athletic and weight-control programs. (It is especially important to involve mothers in diet discussions concerning "her athlete"—she is more apt to think in terms of "well-fed" than lean.) Hand out a simple diet guide—useful until a nutrition training session is held.*
3. Determine and record weights and amount of body fat of each athlete, and set weight goals (5-7 percent of body weight as fat is a minimum goal; 10-12 percent is a good average upper limit for a male in his teens).
4. Conduct an intensive conditioning program for four to six weeks, and plot progress toward goals.
5. Schedule training sessions early for nutrition information. This training could be handled by the home economics staff (foods and nutrition). Let them determine caloric need for each athlete, design a proper diet, and plan menus.
6. Present an exercise-health workshop, which could be set up by the physical education department. The most effective approach to weight reduction and control is a combination diet-exercise program.
7. Keep communication channels open among parents, coaches, and athletes. If the parents are aware of the coach's long range goals, they can do a lot to assist.

*"Ann's Menu Minder" would be helpful for the mother or meal planner—see appendix.

8. Have a "watchdog" program to guard against any drastic measures being used for rapid and excessive weight reduction. Athletes should lose gradually over a period of several weeks. Place constant emphasis on good nutrition related to functions of the body and the dangers of abusing it.
9. Schedule regular workouts during the school holidays to avoid danger of "bouncing" weight.
10. Emphasize enjoyment of the sport engaged in; don't allow development of an attitude of living for the day the season ends. Psychological aspects are a prime consideration of successful athletes.
11. Advise reduction of the caloric intake when training ends. If this isn't done, what usually occurs is a slow increase in the percentage of body fat and a decrease in the percentage of muscle mass—even though body weight may remain relatively stable.
12. Teach lifetime habits of exercise and good nutrition. Ideally, athletes should feel that they are in training all the time.

THE HARDSHIP OF EXTRA FAT

Extra fat is a big problem for many hopeful athletes. For runners and for all too many wrestlers it is a particular concern.

The energy cost for the obese person just to move around is higher than for the person at desirable weight, probably as much as 10 to 15 percent more, depending on the degree of obesity. The overweight individual is under a substantial handicap in any performance associated with locomotion because of a general lack of physical fitness and because of the additional burden of weight. If one is carrying 50 extra pounds, it is almost like carrying a 50-pound bag of flour around all the time. We are expecting our feet and the rest of our body to support all of this extra weight.

Obesity often results in back problems, as well as leg and

foot problems. Balancing all the extra weight as we carry it around throws our bodies out of line, and this leads to poor posture and all the ills associated with poor body alignment. Exercise, such as walking, can be complicated for obese individuals by skin chafing and foot blisters, not to mention difficulties in maintaining body balance and stability.

In overweight athletes a greater load is placed upon the heart and circulatory system, especially when engaged in muscular exertion. For each extra inch around the waist, one mile of blood vessels is added! This means that the heart must work much harder.

The work of breathing also is increased—perhaps by a factor of two—in obese persons. In fact, there is more work for the entire body. As a result, one tires more easily when doing just ordinary routine everyday activities. This may result in the thinner person having all the fun while the obese person just sits.

Sweating is often more profuse in overweight people because the fat below the skin prevents heat from escaping as efficiently as in a person of normal weight.

The more fat one has, the more fat cells there are crying for yet more food. It is a vicious circle of feeding one's fat. Body fat has become one of the main limits on fitness in our over-fed society.

DETERMINING AMOUNT OF BODY FAT

The popular height-weight tables as determined from averaging insurance company statistics of height and weight measurements of individuals of all ages and all sizes do not provide sufficient information to determine how much fat in proportion to body weight a person has. In addition, since the figures are merely averages and because one-fourth of our population is too fat (some even grossly obese), the weight figures tend to be higher than they actually should be. Reducing the weight statistics by 10 percent would be an appropriate correction for above-average weight.

In 1940, just prior to World War II, Dr. Albert Behnke, Jr., a recognized authority on body composition, made detailed measurements of size, shape, and structure of 25 professional football players. He compared these measurements to the military standards at that time. A person whose body weight was 15 percent above the "average weight according to height" as determined from the chart developed from insurance company statistics was designated overweight and rejected by the military.

When he applied these so-called standard weights to the football players, he found that 17 out of 25 were classified as too fat and unfit for military service. But, on more careful examination, he discovered that 11 of the 17 actually had a relatively small percentage of body fat. The extra weight was due primarily to their large muscular development.

Dr. Behnke's findings clearly illustrated that the popular height-weight tables provide little information with regard to the *composition* of an individual's body weight. An athlete's extra weight may consist of a considerable amount of muscle mass. As a consequence, the use of height-weight tables can be quite misleading for the person who wants to know, "How fat am I?"

There are a number of different methods to assess the ideal weight and amount of fat of athletes. Some are very simple to apply while others take complicated, expensive equipment and much technical skill. (The latter will not be discussed here.) All techniques are designed to measure the amount of body fat in comparison to the lean body mass that an individual possesses. The lean body mass includes the muscle, bone, and organ tissues. The word "subcutaneous" is used to describe the fat that is situated directly beneath the skin.

The skin-fold test for subcutaneous fat gives us a rough estimate of body condition. One simple rule of thumb is to pinch the skin on the forehead at the outer, upper area above the eye and compare its thickness to the skin fold over the abdomen and over the back of the arm of the athlete. A well-conditioned athlete will have approximately the same thickness of subcutaneous fat in all three places. This is a rough estimate, and it would be helpful to have a pair of skin-fold calipers and a conversion table to use as a guideline.* The subcutaneous fat on the back of the arm over the triceps in a conditioned athlete should average 6 to 8 millimeters or slightly less (approximately ¼ inch). The pinch test can apply to non-athletes as well as athletes. If we feel more than an inch of flesh between our thumb and forefinger, we are carrying excess weight.

Another simple test is the ruler test: the athlete lies flat on his back in a relaxed state. Since the surface of the abdomen between the ribs and the pubis is normally flat or slightly concave, a ruler placed on the abdomen parallel with the vertical axis of the body should touch both ribs and pelvic area.

The beltline test (specifically for males) involves measurement of the girth of the chest (at the level of the nipples) and the abdomen (at the level of the navel). The chest should be larger than the abdomen by several inches.

DETERMINING PROPER BODY WEIGHT

Proper body weight is unique to each individual, based on body makeup and the physical activity to be undertaken, and there is no simple way to determine one's best weight. The best weight represents maximum strength with minimum extra baggage (fat).

An athlete needs to be concerned about his proper weight, but besides being concerned about reducing excess fat, he is equally interested in increasing muscle mass. When an athlete exercises, he loses fat and develops muscle mass, and this will change his weight and physique.

Proper weight is important to the athlete, not only to the

*Dr. Jean Mayer in *Overweight: Causes, Cost, and Control,* 1968, reported that the most practical method to measure the fat content of the body is by use of calipers to measure skin-folds. He found that the triceps skin-fold is the easiest to measure and also the most representative of total body fatness.

extent that it affects his performance but also in the way he feels mentally and the way he looks and feels physically. Also, proper weight is a factor in the athlete's susceptibility to disease and injury.

During the past fifty years many laboratory procedures have been developed to analyze the body in relation to its three major structural components: fat, muscle, and bone. Several methods have been used, including skin-fold thickness, anthropometric measurement, body densitometry, total body potassium levels, and radial-ulnar diameter measurements. There is a need for a simple but meaningful method of assessing body composition, including the amount of adipose tissue (fat).

In determining proper weight for athletes, we've discovered that the usual height-weight charts are not very useful since the athlete is concerned not only with total weight but also the muscle-fat composition of that weight. Football players, as Dr. Behnke found, frequently would be termed overweight (if not obese) according to height-weight charts. But in sports where muscular development is a significant factor in the training process, the body weight of participating athletes may seem very high although the fat percentage is quite acceptable.

In determining proper weight it is important to know what percentage of total fat is desirable. The ideal percentage of fat for the American non-athlete is now considered to be about 16 percent. A typical 16-year-old high school boy who weighs about 155 pounds can be expected to have body fat amounting to 15 to 17 percent of his total weight. However, a well-conditioned athlete would have his weight down to include only 5 to 8 percent body fat, and a wrestler trimmed down to only 5 percent body fat is probably at the lowest level possible for performance with stamina.

Each person seems to have a biological limit below which he or she cannot reduce body weight and still maintain good health. This lower limit is referred to as lean body weight.

To determine proper body weight, then, the amount of body fat should be determined. The simplest and most accurate method of estimating the fat is through measurement of skin-fold thickness. This requires a pair of skin-fold calipers and a conversion table with which to estimate the percent of total body weight represented by fat tissue. These measurements can be used to establish the minimum (and most effective) weight for each athlete.

A hopeful athlete should participate in an intensive conditioning program for at least four to six weeks. At the end of this conditioning period, determine weight each day before eating breakfast but after urinating. Consider this weight the athlete's most effective level for the season (unless skin-fold tests show that body fat still is excessive).

The athlete who is functioning with a normal level of body fluid, optimal muscle mass, and no excessive body fat is very likely to be at his most effective weight.

WEIGHT REDUCTION

What you eat shows. Excess weight is caused by eating in excess of what your body needs.

Weight reduction requires recognizing excess fat and determining to do something about it. Your doctor and your coach can help you assess the fat content of your body and determine what your weight should be. All athletes should be made aware of their percentage of body fat so that they can make a sincere effort to lose the excess.

Food Intake Must Be Planned

A weight reduction program must be carefully planned, and the athlete should understand what foods the body needs and in what amounts. Controlling the appetite is a necessary and effective way to reduce weight. When hunger urges you to eat, curb the appetite by drinking water instead.

Wide variations in individuals, not only in physical structure but in mental attitude and the ability for self-discipline, make it difficult to plan toward a specific percentage of weight loss.

If weight is lost gradually through a properly planned diet and no more than 8-10 percent of body weight is lost over a period of several weeks, an athlete should suffer no ill effects.

If we want to reduce, we must run a calorie deficit. To lose 1 pound a week, we need to subtract 500 calories a day from our maintenance diet. A maintenance diet provides the total number of calories a day to keep one at an even weight. The total can be determined approximately by multiplying weight in pounds by 15 (for those who are moderately active).

Under no circumstances should a hardworking athlete have his caloric intake limited to less than 1,000 calories a day on a regular basis. No harm is done by having to miss a meal occasionally, but if the caloric intake is much less than basal requirements over a long period of weight reduction, the loss in weight will result from deterioration of muscles as well as from loss of fat.

A healthy adult can fast for two weeks and suffer no permanent ill effects, but it should be done only under medical supervision. (See later discussions on ketosis in Chapter 15, and fasting in Chapter 13.) During starvation, the exhaustive time for body carbohydrate is less than one day whereas protein and fat can provide sufficient reserves for up to forty days.

When an individual fasts, he may lose weight rapidly. The glucose and glycogen stores are utilized during the first day; a large quantity of water is also lost. The individual can lose close to 3 pounds in one day of complete fasting if he has expended approximately 3,500 calories. He would lose 1 pound of body tissue and approximately 2 pounds of water.

After the first day, protein and fat supply the energy for bodily functions. Without carbohydrate to use as energy, for example, some of the protein would be converted into glucose to be used by the central nervous system since the brain requires nourishment in order to function. During prolonged starvation, the brain begins to utilize ketone bodies, intermediate products of fat metabolism, for its energy source.

In a resting adult about 1,600 calories per day, the basal metabolism rate, will be used. Protein will supply about 250 of the calories and fat 1,350. Weight loss without exercise, relying on starvation, will result in a wasting of muscle tissue. Starvation and dehydration can jeopardize health.

Remember to eat a variety of foods but eat small or very small portions, depending on how much weight there is to be lost and how fast you want to lose it. A reducing diet should have the following: no less than 12-14 percent protein, no more than about 30 percent fat (keep down the saturated fat), and the remainder (about 50 percent) in carbohydrates with sucrose held to a low level. Eliminate as much fat as you can—eat lean meats and fish. Use lots of vegetables and fewer fruits because there are more calories in fruits. Substitute grapefruit for orange juice to minimize calories.

Eat regular meals—three a day or five or whatever, but establish regularity. Avoid snacking. Eating a good breakfast is *important*. Drink plenty of liquids to protect the fluid balance of your body and to help your body carry away wastes. Water also helps alleviate hunger pangs. Keep a record of weight loss; a graph-type chart lends encouragement, especially if one is making steady progress. (It is a gentle reminder—if one is not.)

(See "Liquid Protein" in Chapter 22 for information on a current reducing fad.)

An Exercise Program is Necessary

It is usually not very successful to try to lose weight by calorie deficit only since there is a definite limit to the nourishment your body can do without. If one is trying to lose about four pounds a week, a good exercise program will be mandatory.

A combination of exercise and reduction of food consumption is the best way to reduce. Weight lost by exercise is more apt to be permanent than that lost only by limiting calories. Exercise also has concomitant benefits on the cardiovascular system.

In walking, the average person uses approximately 100

calories a mile; thus, one must walk 35 miles in order to lose 1 pound of weight! But 2 miles a day will result in a loss of slightly less than 2 pounds a month. If the individual can train to running 5 miles a day, 1 pound a week can be lost. Over a year's time, the loss can be substantial. Overweight people will expend even more energy while exercising; hence their exercise will be more effective in losing weight.

Many people try to reduce by spot reduction without realizing that spot reduction is not possible. We can exercise specific areas to solidify certain muscle tissue that underlies the excessive adipose tissue, but for the most part, we cannot control where the fat comes off.

Hopeful athletes have been known to think they can change fat into muscle, without realizing that although fat and muscle both contain water, fat, and protein, their composition is very different. A pound of fat has 3,500 calories while a pound of muscle contains only 600 calories. Most muscle is water, whereas fatty tissue is mainly fat. One must exercise first to burn up the fat surplus, and then exercise more in the specific area where you want muscle to be built. Intensive use of a part of the body builds and strengthens and firms muscle tissue in that part, but fat doesn't change directly into muscle.

Special Weight Problems of Wrestlers

Wrestling is one of the few sports sanctioned by scholastic and collegiate athletic groups that regulates competition by body weight classes, and in some states individuals must be "certified" for specific weight classes by weighing in at designated time periods, usually several days before the season begins.

Athletes, and particularly wrestlers, should be encouraged to keep their weight within two to four pounds of their certified weight throughout the season. Let a wrestler go up in weight to fill a weight class, especially if he is still growing, but he should not be encouraged to go down in weight if his body fat is minimum for him.

According to coaches and professional trainers, most really

well-conditioned male athletes have their body fat down to levels of 5 to 7 percent of body weight.

Wrestlers wishing to cut down to another weight class should do it over an extended period of time. Set goals, such as three pounds each week, and attain desired weight reduction by cutting food intake and increasing exercise.

Coaches of grade school and high school wrestlers (and other athletes, too) could eliminate a big problem with mothers if they would plan to "build up" their aspiring young athletes with good diet and muscle-building programs rather than taking them down one or two weight classes. But if an athlete is considerably overweight, a good weight-reduction plan should allow the athlete to drop to a lower weight class. (In that case, the coach should confer with the parents of the athlete so they can see the value of a weight-reduction plan.)

Coaches suggest that the best time to trim off excess weight is in the off-season months. Then the athlete can report for training trim and fit!

Homeostasis Principle

The tendency of an organism to maintain a uniform and beneficial physiological stability within and between its parts is called homeostasis. The individual who has achieved a long-dreamed-of weight-reduction goal will be comforted to know that if he can maintain the new weight for a period of time, at least a few months, it will be easier to continue maintenance of the new weight because the body by then will have established an equilibrium within the new weight limit. Once a weight has been *established*, it is more difficult to achieve either a weight loss or gain than when the weight is changing; the body's tendency is to resist change whether that change is a desirable norm or not.

If one has achieved a new weight, it is good to be reminded of the "homeostasis" principle" and to do all in one's power to preserve the new weight for several weeks while the body is making the adjustment.

Crash Weight Cutting

There are several ways used by athletes to "make weight" in a hurry. None is advised. Drastic, quick-loss schemes often are self-defeating and can result in physical damage.

Water is the most easily manipulated factor to use for acute weight loss, but it is probably the most dangerous to manipulate. Water restriction should not be practiced because all body processes depend on a supply of water.

The use of "sweating" is a common practice; this includes taking long saunas or working out in rubber suits to lose body fluid, sometimes resulting in severe dehydration.

Body fluid weight is much easier to lose than body fat, and this is the course that many athletes and coaches follow without realizing the possible dangers inherent in it. Body fluid is not excess weight, and it is important to keep it in good balance. Cells are bathed in fluid that is in a delicate electrolyte balance for movement of nutrients and transfer of gases in the tissues. If there is rapid or prolonged dehydration, the electrolyte balance is upset, leading to weakness, muscular uncoordination, neuralgic disturbances, stress on the cardiovascular system, and lack of mental alertness. For best physical health, it is best not to upset the vital body-fluid balance.

Starvation or semi-starvation is practiced by some athletes in hopes of losing weight quickly. On a diet inadequate in energy to meet body needs, the body constantly is burning some of its stored fat. Because fats are incompletely oxidized due to limited carbohydrates available (when the athlete is eating nothing), fatty acids accumulate, causing an uncomfortable acidosis, or ketosis, condition. To avoid this, a small amount of carbohydrate must be included in the reducing diet. A minimum of 50-70 calories of carbohydrate a day is needed to help combat the threat of ketosis on an extreme reducing binge. Citrus fruits, dark green and yellow vegetables, and skim milk are carbohydrates that should be included in the reducing diet, plus a serving of whole-grain bread or cereal.

Vitamins and minerals, important to the diet, are included in these foods.

Athletes sometimes resort to the use of a diuretic, a substance that will increase the secretion of urine by the kidneys. But increased urine flow results also in the forced excretion of electrolytes, particularly the sodium and potassium electrolytes. The use of diuretics in medical practice is justified sometimes when it is important to remove excess fluids, but their use by athletes as a means of reducing weight is not approved.

Another extreme measure sometimes applied is the use of a cathartic. A cathartic is a substance used to remove food residue and water from the intestinal tract. This removal action leads to water loss as well as electrolyte depletion, especially of the sodium and potassium electrolytes. Potassium is necessary for muscle function, and the "washed out" feeling following the use of a cathartic is due largely to the loss of potassium and body fluid.

The use of diuretics and cathartics are methods of weight reduction that disturb the acid-base as well as the water-electrolyte balance of the body. They have no place in athletic weight-reduction programs.

"Spitting" (or regurgitation) is another "weight-making" practice. It is probably the most widely used and the least harmful. Repulsive perhaps, but it is practiced. A danger is that performance may be affected adversely by the loss of potassium present in the digestive juices of saliva.

The athlete who does not keep his weight within limits and then totally starves himself for a few days, along with total dehydration to make a specific weight, is abusing himself. When tournament time comes along, he cannot last through the days of competition.

An athlete who is constantly hungry, dehydrated, uncomfortable, tired, and has depleted his needed energy reservoir is comparable to an injured athlete. If an athlete is continually going over his weight class, he probably is in the wrong weight grouping.

In order to compete, a wrestler may be under special pressure to meet a designated weight, and this sometimes leads to problems both for him and the coach. But the athlete himself should bear a large part of the blame if he is engaging in dangerous "making weight" practices. Many times they are of his own doing. It may be lack of knowledge of the dangers involved or lack of enough self-discipline to eat properly. Hopefully, this discussion will discourage those poor practices.

SUMMARY

There are no short cuts to weight reduction and weight control. It is plain hard work to get rid of body fat. There is no magic way—we simply must eat fewer calories than we burn up and then burn up some more by engaging in exercise. Patience and discipline are further requirements for successful fat removal. It is easier to *keep it off* than to *take it off!*

If losing weight permanently is one's goal, something more than just a change in diet is needed. One will need a new way of eating and a change in *why, what,* and *how much* one eats—a plan that will help for a lifetime. The more limited one's calorie intake, the more important it is that one plans meals carefully to include the essential nutrients each day.* An exercise program should be included in a weight-reduction plan, but exercise only is an inefficient way to lose weight compared to calorie restriction.

Medical and nutrition consultants believe that the best way to lose weight is by long-term calorie restriction, regular and well-balanced meals, and moderate to brisk exercise. For *permanent* results, overweight people must change their life-styles permanently!

Once an athlete has arrived at his desired weight, he should stay there! Keep in training all the time. Counteract the tendency to overeat on weekends and vacations.

---

*See appendix for information on "Ann's Menu Minder" kit for nutrition information and menu suggestions.

REFERENCES FOR FURTHER READING
Books

Gregg, W.H. *Physical Fitness through Sports and Nutrition.* New York: Scribner's, 1975.

Katch, F.I., and W.D. McArdle. *Nutrition, Weight Control and Exercise.* Boston: Houghton-Mifflin, 1977.

Mayer, Jean. *Human Nutrition.* Springfield, Illinois: Charles C. Thomas, 1972.

O'Shea, J.P. *Scientific Principles and Methods of Strength Fitness.* Rev. ed. Reading, Massachusetts: Addison-Wesley, 1969.

Wilmore, J.H. *Athletic Training and Physical Fitness.* Boston: Allyn and Bacon, 1976.

Periodicals

Evans, R.I., and Y.Hall. "Social Psychological Perspective on Motivating Changes in Eating Behavior," *J.Amer. Dietet. A.,* 72:378 (April 1978).

Hansen, Norman C. "Wrestling with 'Making Weight,'" *The Physician and Sportsmedicine,* 6: 107-1 (April 1978).

Kirshenbaum, J. "Pricking Up Their Ears; Lactic Acid Blood Testing to Determine Most Efficient Training Pace," *Sports Illustrated,* 47:94+ (October 31, 1977).

Krzywicki, H.J., G.M. Ward, D.P. Rahman, R.A. Nelson and C.F. Consolazio. "A Comparison of Methods for Estimating Human Body Composition," *Am. J. Clin. Nutr.* 27: 1380 (December 1974).

Mahoney, M.J., and A.W. Caggiula. "Applying Behavioral Methods to Nutrition Counseling," *J. Am. Deitet, A.,* 72-372 (April 1978).

Nutrition Reviews "Nature of Weight Loss During Short-Term Dieting," 36:72-4 (March 1978).

Scrimshaw, Nevin S. "Through a Glass Darkly: Discerning the Practical Implications of Human Dietary Protein— Energy Interrelationships," *Nutrition Reviews,* 35: 321-37 (December 1977).

part 3

Eating for Performance

10

The Daily Food Intake

Food is the fuel that makes possible all of the body's activities. There is little evidence that athletes have special nutritional requirements, but some knowledge of what foods are needed, what nutrients, what combinations of them, and in what amounts can be significant in the development and functioning of the successful athlete.

Food alone doesn't make the champion athlete, but the performance of an athlete is enhanced by good nutrition. Conversely, performance is seriously hampered by an improper diet since the lack of some foods, both as to kind and amount, can reduce the efficiency of the body to less than maximal.

The basic nutritional principles described in this book apply to both the athlete and the non-athlete, but the athlete will need more calories for his increased energy expenditure.

During training the athlete should consume his extra calories in the form of milk, meat, vegetables, and grain products. This will satisfy his increased demand for carbohydrates, proteins, and regulatory vitamins and minerals.

Good nutrition promotes the ability of the body to work efficiently and develop fully, thus paving the way to success in athletic or other endeavors.

DAILY FOOD SCORE CHART

Do you have any idea how much or how little you eat? To check, use the Daily Food Score Chart to evaluate the distribution of foods within the daily intake. For a week keep an accurate daily meal record, recording the amount and type of food ingested for breakfast, lunch, dinner, and all snacks during the day.

By using this chart you will become more aware of the foods needed and the so-called "ideal" number of servings; it is a good way to check how you measure up in eating habits.

Most athletes need much the same kinds of foods as other people, but the athlete who is quite active will need more carbohydrates and fats for energy. The bread and cereal group (carbohydrates) and some fats supply good sources of energy; increase the number of servings in these groups for added calories. If an athlete is extremely active, increase the number and size of servings in all the food groups in order to meet the needed requirement of nutrients. Use cracked-grain cereal or enriched grain products for increased nutrition. Sugar products, such as candy and carbonated beverages, should be limited (or even eliminated) in the diet.

A BALANCED DIET

All nutrients in foods work as teams in the body; that is why it is important to eat a well-balanced diet. Thus, the nutrients from some foods will be in the body together with nutrients from other foods, and they can function as a team. Imagine some members of a basketball squad practicing when the others are sleeping—the team would never be able to work

DAILY FOOD SCORE CHART (check your daily servings)

Food Group	*Meals*					
Refer to "Ideal" column for number of daily servings for good nutrition. List the servings of each food group you ate ... in the "Meals" columns. Totals will indicate your eating habits.	*B r e a k* *f a s t*	*L u n c h*	*D i n n e r*	*S n a c k s*	*T o t a l s*	*I d e a l*
FRUITS & VEGETABLES Fruit: citrus (vitamin C)						1
Fruit: deep yellow Vegetables: deep yellow, dark green, leafy						1 every other day
Fruit: non-citrus; Potatoes and other vegetables not included in above						2 or 3 or more
MILK PRODUCTS						4
MEAT GROUP						2
BREADS & CEREALS						4
FATS & OILS						1-2 tbsp.
SUGAR & STUFF						0

Suggestion: A loose-leaf notebook may be the best place to record the food eaten during the trial period of examining your daily food habits. Record food eaten, and each evening check with this chart to determine if you have eaten foods during the day that are needed by your body. Or are you eating a lot of "extras" that merely add calories and possible fat?

together; they must all be present at the same time to succeed as a successful team.

When our diet provides for the body's energy, growth, and maintenance needs, it is said to be a "balanced diet." It is important for the athlete to develop an awareness of a balanced diet and the special requirements of his body because of the extra energy needed in athletic training.

We are fortunate to have a vast variety of foods, but since science has discovered that the body needs some 50 nutrients and *no one* food contains all known nutrients, some knowledge and planning are necessary to meet the daily food requirement. The grouping of food into general categories of fruits and vegetables, milk products, meat or meat alternates, breads and cereals, and fats and oils helps to clarify what our body needs. Learn the food groupings and how much you need of those foods each day; discover all the variety of possibilities in each group—eating doesn't need to be monotonous.

Making food choices in meal planning can be a pretty complicated business, but we will simplify meal planning as much as possible in hopes that the athlete will be encouraged to tackle the process. It is the best way of assuring good nutrition.

From the Daily Food Guide, select important vitamin- and mineral-packed fruits and vegetables. One serving of citrus fruits or tomatoes, which are good sources of vitamin C,

DAILY FOOD GUIDE

Fruits & Vegetables
Citrus (High in vitamin C): 1 serving each day
Dark Green, Leafy, or **Deep Yellow** (high in vitamin A): 1 serving every other day
Other Fruits & Vegetables:
Select 2 or more servings from this group to make a total of 4 or more each day

Milk Products
Children: . . . . 3-4 cups
Teenagers: . . . . 4 cups
Adults: . . . . 2 cups

Meat Group
(Includes eggs, cheese, fish, poultry, dry peas, beans, and nuts)
2 (or more) servings

Breads and Cereals
4 (or more) servings

Fats & Oils
1 to 2 tablespoons

Sugar and Stuff
Keep to a minimum

DAILY MENU PATTERN

Breakfast
Citrus Fruit
Hot or Cold Cereal
Bread (with spread)
Eggs and Meat
(if desired)
Beverage

Lunch
Soup
Sandwich
Salad
(or relishes)
Dessert
Beverage

Dinner
Meat
(or alternate)
Potatoes
(or cereal product)
Vegetables
(green or yellow)
Salad
(fruit or vegetable)
Bread
Dessert
Beverage

SAMPLE DAILY MENU

Breakfast
Orange Juice
Hot Cereal
Toast, Jelly
Beverage

Lunch
Tomato Soup
Cheese Sandwich (toasted)
Celery & Carrot Sticks
Banana
Milk

Dinner
Roast Beef (lean)
Baked Squash or Potatoes
Tossed Salad & Oil Dressing
Whole Wheat Rolls & Butter
Fruit Cup
Beverage

should be eaten every day. Other choices can include oranges, grapefruit, cantaloupe, strawberries, broccoli, and green cabbage.

A dark green, leafy, or deep yellow vegetable should be eaten four or five times a week for vitamin A. (If it is easier to remember a vitamin A vegetable or fruit every other day, that is fine.) Other fruits and vegetables, including potatoes, whether they are fresh, frozen, or canned, should be in the diet for variety as well as for good sources of vitamins, minerals, and roughage. One should have a total of four or more vegetables and fruits each day; the servings can be small if one is watching weight or larger if additional calories are desired. Vegetables contain more vitamins and minerals than most fruits (except for citrus), and they usually have fewer calories. From the milk products group, an athlete should select at least four servings of milk a day; this can include ice cream, cheeses, or milk in soups, custards, puddings, or combined with other foods (as on cereal). If weight is a problem, drink skim milk—you'll get the nutrients without the fat; be sure it is fortified with vitamins A and D.

If an athlete eliminates dairy products from his diet, getting enough calcium is a real problem since dairy products are the principal sources of calcium. Fair calcium sources are nuts, legumes, dark green leafy vegetables, canned salmon and sardines (fish with bones are a good source).

Foods in the meat (or meat alternate) group should be eaten twice a day to supply the protein requirement. Animal products such as meat, fish, poultry, cheese, and eggs are excellent sources of the "essential" amino acids, but dried beans or peas and peanut butter are also good sources of high-quality protein. Eggs and meat, in addition to having value as protein, are good sources of iron and some of the B vitamins. Athletes not eating animal protein can rely on vegetable protein, dairy products, and cereal grains eaten in combinations that make complete proteins.

In the bread and cereal groups, four servings a day are desirable. Choices may be made from breads, cooked and ready-to-eat cereals, pasta products such as enriched macaroni and spaghetti, rice, and baked goods made from whole-grain or enriched flours. The bread and cereal group is a good source of energy as well as B vitamins and some protein. Bread and milk or cereal and milk consumed together make a complete protein.

Include a little vegetable oil (containing linoleic acid) each day; at least a tablespoon or two of an oil dressing can serve as this source. Vegetable cellulose (fiber) is present in cereal grains and in many vegetables; eating these raw or cooked is an aid in the digestive tract.

BREAKFAST AND ITS IMPORTANCE

Since breakfast marks the end of an overnight fast, it is thought to be the most important meal of the day. It is especially important if the athlete participates in training activities in the late afternoon, which is the universal training time for almost all school athletes.

Research is limited as to the effect that breakfast has upon physical performance, but enough study has been done to determine that the omission of breakfast usually results in a lower total work output. However, it is surprising that no particular difference in work output is noticed when comparing the benefits of a breakfast of carbohydrates, consisting of fruit, cereals, toast, and milk, to a breakfast featuring protein, with bacon and eggs substituted for the cereal. The important thing is to eat a breakfast consisting of good wholesome food.

We are aware that there are individuals who don't feel hungry at breakfast time. These individuals should try the following: refrain from eating solid foods just before going to bed, perform some light exercise after arising in the morning, and drink a sizable quantity of milk. The stomach soon will become accustomed to the food intake and begin to require it.

For optimum energy and minimum fat storage, 35 to 40 percent of total calories consumed daily should be eaten at breakfast. Then eat a moderate noon meal and a light evening meal. If the athlete plans on 3,600 calories a day, a breakfast allotment of about 1,350 calories would be about right.

Breakfast should contain both protein and carbohydrate foods, and the carbohydrates should be predominately starch in content rather than sugar in order to maintain a slower release of blood sugar over a longer period of time. Sugar is a fast-spurt source of energy, which is desirable at times for an athlete, but sugar in the meal is not as long-lasting as starch, and the individual often will feel the need for snacking between meals.

Breakfast is a good time to satisfy the vitamin C requirements for the day with orange, grapefruit, or other vitamin C fruit. Inclusion of eggs is a personal preference. Some doctors suggest limiting eggs in breakfast menus because of the cholesterol problem; others reason that the risk is worth the benefits because eggs are such a rich-in-iron food and the egg white is pure protein (no fat). Besides, if the athlete is extremely active, there may be less chance of cholesterol build-up. Hot cereal or granola is a good breakfast food for all ages. Cereal and milk, consumed together, make a complete protein, which is low in fat and relatively inexpensive. Remember that bacon and sausages are high in fat; if your food budget and your protein-carbohydrate calorie allowance will permit, you may include them, but if you eat cereal and milk together, you do not need bacon, eggs, or sausage for protein.

Breakfasts are often a problem for teenagers. They sometimes are bored with the same old thing! There is no reason why hamburgers should not be acceptable in the morning. Hamburger is a good substitute for eggs and bacon, and buns replace the usual toast.

Early settlers in New England cut slices of mince and apple pie for their early morning meal. Custard or even pumpkin pie is a good way to create variety with eggs in the morning.

Apple, carrot, or fruit cake with little or no icing contains more nutritive value than a sweet roll. Fruit breads are also excellent breakfast breads.

BEVERAGES—ATHLETE'S CHOICE
Milk

There has been a tendency for coaches to restrict the consumption of milk for athletes during training and immediately preceding athletic competition. Varied reasons have been advanced for this restriction, including the supposition that milk contributes to the development of "cottonmouth."

"Cottonmouth" is a dryness and discomfort (fuzzy feeling) in the mouth due to a decrease in activity of salivary glands. It is not affected by the kind of food eaten (or by milk drunk) before an athletic event. The saliva flow is decreased with increasing amounts of perspiration and reduced water content of the body and also can be influenced by one's emotional state. If tension causes the mouth of the player to feel dry, chewing gum often is helpful; drinking water or sucking on ice also can help.

Some athletes and coaches feel that milk decreases speed of movement and "cuts wind," but that is not true. There is no difference in training response or in performance when milk is either included or excluded from the diet. If an athlete likes milk and wants it in his pregame meal, there is no justifiable reason to eliminate it.

Restriction of milk in the diet should not be made without a particular reason, but we should be aware that milk sugar is not well digested by some racial groups. For example, sometimes black athletes have difficulty digesting milk. In some, milk causes gases, diarrhea, and cramps. One of the most frequent causes of problems in the digestion of milk products is the lack of an intestinal enzyme, lactase, which is essential for the proper breakdown of milk.

When milk products are eliminated from the diet, nutrients such as calcium and riboflavin can easily fall below recommended levels. The team of calcium, phosphorous, protein, and vitamins C and D builds bones. Milk and milk products provide most of the calcium for good bone growth.

Fruit Juice

Fruit juices are highly recommended and should be selected in preference to soft drinks as a general habit, but the athlete should be aware of the calories in fruit juices and realize that there is no need to drink a *surplus* of juice. The body can utilize only so much of the vitamins and minerals contained in any food, and after one has satisfied the mineral and vitamin requirements, it is a waste of money and good food to eat or drink a surplus. It also adds calories that probably are not needed. It is better to drink only the fruit juices to supply vitamins and minerals, the needs of the body, and to drink water for the remaining fluid needs.

The natural sugars in oranges, apples, and many other fruit juices make them slightly higher in total sugar content than a bottle of cola, but there is an important difference: fruit juices offer other nutrients besides calories. Try to satisfy your craving for sweets with fresh or dried fruits and fruit juices.

Coffee (Caffeine)

Caffeine is an alkaloid, a nitrogenous organic base found in a large number of plants throughout the world: the coffee bean came from Arabia, the tea leaf from China, the kola nut from West Africa, and the cocoa bean from Mexico. They all contain caffeine, a natural component of each plant's bean, leaf, or nut.

Caffeine is a popular, short-term stimulant that fits the definition of a drug. Caffeine is absorbed rapidly and reaches peak levels in the body within about an hour after ingestion: within a short time it enters all organs and tissues. It is a stimulant to the central nervous system and affects the cerebral cortex, medulla, and spinal cord. Even a small to moderate amount of caffeine received by the central nervous system results in increased alertness and a reduction of fatigue. This is a short-term effect, and the exact mechanism by which fatigue is allayed is not clearly understood. It is thought that the individual's perception of fatigue is prevented by caffeine's action on the brain, and the ability for increased capacity to work is the result. Caffeine also stimulates the cardiac muscle, increasing the strength of its contractions. Also, in moderate to large doses caffeine causes an increase in the rate and depth of breathing through its action on the medulla.

It is the caffeine in coffee that triggers the release of some stored body energy, and this action puts more sugar into the bloodstream. We say we "get a lift"—and we do; but after about three hours we feel a "let down"—fatigue, with decreased efficiency and alertness. The stimulating effect of caffeine in the blood plasma and organs has worn off.

Caffeine is touted as the best easily available and acceptable drug to aid athletic performance because temporarily it can delay fatigue, increase alertness, and influence motor ability. If the athlete feels tired or nervous and is in need of a little aid to increase efficiency, a cup of coffee may provide the "lift" that he wants. (A cup of coffee contains approximately 85 mg of caffeine.)

Tolerance to caffeine varies widely among individuals. A normal person can tolerate the amount of caffeine in coffee without apparent discomfort. Caffeine is not adaptive, that is, regular consumption does not diminish its stimulant effects. People who drink lots of coffee from age 20 on, may experience some difficulty with caffeine after age 40. They would not experience the caffeine effects if they switched to decaffeinated coffee, but the volatile oil in the coffee bean (which gives most of the flavor and color) is still present, and this oil is an irritant to some people.

The chronic effects of a long-time habit of drinking five or more cups of coffee a day may include irritation of mucous membranes, digestive disturbances, loss of sleep, increased nervous irritability, increased blood pressure, palpitation of the heart, muscular tremors, and even peptic ulcer distress. High levels of caffeine do become toxic, but no deaths from caffeine poisoning have ever been reported, and there is no evidence to show that *small amounts* of this beverage are harmful in an athlete's diet. There appears, also, to be no particular reason to either advocate the use of a mild stimulant, such as coffee, or to suggest complete avoidance of it.

Caffeine is widely used for its stimulant properties in beverages and in over-the-counter drugs and prescriptions. Caffeine is preferred and accepted as a safe stimulant.

Tea

The effect of a cup of tea is similar to that of coffee. One cup of tea has about one-half to two-thirds as much caffeine as a cup of coffee. In addition, it contains tannic acid, which retards digestion when the brew is strong. However, most people do not like strong tea, and many people like their tea half-and-half with milk. Tea with a little honey is enjoyed as a stimulant by some athletes.

Besides caffeine and tannic acid, tea also contains an ingredient called theophylline, which is used as a coronary dilator.

Cola

An 8-ounce bottle of cola contains about 100 calories and very few, if any, nutrients. Many parents do not allow their children to drink coffee, but 3 cola drinks can equal the caffeine in a cup of coffee. The drinking of colas has increased, and the consumption of milk and fruit juice has decreased. Colas may be used in moderation if they do not replace other liquid foods such as milk and fruit juice. Remember, soft drinks are 10 to 15 percent sugar (except for the sugar-free kind).

Cola drinks do little for an athlete except to add liquid and "empty" calories without contributing any valuable nutrients for body building and repair. Young athletes have the chance to develop good lifelong eating habits without the "sugar dependencies" of our present habits.

It is suggested that an athlete desiring to use a beverage such as coffee, tea, or cola as a stimulant should plan his use of these beverages immediately prior to an event. However, 3 or 4 hours later, if the athlete still is performing, efficiency could be noticeably impaired. Thus, unless one plans the time-release factors of a "lift" within 30 minutes and a "let down" after 3 or 4 hours, the use of any beverage with caffeine is not advised before competition.

11

Eating Schedule for the Athlete

AFTER-SCHOOL WORKOUTS

The most important meal of the day is *breakfast* if an athlete participates in training activities in late afternoon. See "Breakfast and Its Importance" in Chapter 10 for foods to include. About 35 to 40 percent of total daily calories should be consumed at this meal.

Lunch should consist of easily digested foods—about 30 to 35 percent of total caloric intake should occur at this noon-day meal. Plan a high proportion of proteins and carbohydrates; carbohydrates can be easily-digested fruits and fruit juices; proteins may be milk puddings. Also include low-cellulose salads such as fruit and cottage cheese and cooked vegetables with little or no fat. Protein foods at lunch may be hearty sandwiches with meat and cheese plus milk soups.

Evening meal should ideally be the lightest of all—25 to 30 percent of total daily caloric intake. The protein content should be high, with a smaller proportion of the more easily digested fats. Salads with a high cellulose content (lettuce, cabbage, etc.) and salad oil dressings should be eaten at this meal. This provides important roughage to aid regular bowel movement. Remember: excess carbohydrates, fats, and protein eaten at dinner time and not used for energy purposes eventually are deposited in the body as subcutaneous fat.

MORNING WORKOUTS

Breakfast should be easily digested protein and high carbohydrate foods, including citrus fruit. Fats should be kept to a minimum at this meal eaten before practice. Decrease the food calorie intake by 5 to 10 percent from that of afternoon trainers.

Lunch should be the heaviest meal of the day for an athlete working out in the morning. It should be increased in total calorie intake by 5 to 10 percent so that it is larger than breakfast. Include foods of protein, carbohydrate, and fat content. Lunch should be similar to the breakfast pattern of the athlete who trains in late afternoon.

Dinner should consist of easily digested foods with a high proportion of proteins and carbohydrates, including cooked vegetables, fruits, puddings, soups, and sandwiches. This meal is similar to the lunch pattern of the afternoon trainer.

GOOD EATING PRACTICES

Some athletes feel they can maintain a more even energy level by eating less at each meal but eating more often; instead of three regular meals they have five or six small ones.

Meals should be eaten at regular hours. If meals are consistently missed or eaten at different times each day, there is an inhibitory reflex put out by the brain, the secretion of digestive juices is slowed down or halted, and appetite is weakened and in many cases lost.

An athlete who is watching weight, besides eating regular

meals should learn to eat slowly. Twenty minutes is required for the brain to send a message that the need for food has been satisfied. If one is eating hurriedly, one will have over-eaten long before the message has been relayed from the brain.

Important to remember: food eaten early in the day is more apt to be used as energy; food eaten at the end of the day is more apt to be stored as fat. There is no suggested length for a rest period following eating and before resuming exercise; it will vary with the type and amount of food eaten, state of mind of the athlete, and the type of activity in which he engages.

The energy-releasing processes for any food are elaborate. Food remains in the stomach from one and one-half to six hours. Liquid meals and carbohydrate-rich meals are in the stomach the shortest length of time: one and one-half to three hours. Meals high in protein and fat take longer to process— up to six hours. Food then passes from the stomach to the small intestine, where the digestive process requires an additional three to four hours before the cells receive benefit or the body receives energy from that particular meal. An athlete eating breakfast in the morning hours will benefit from that meal during afternoon practice.

MINIMUM DAILY FOOD LINE-UP
FOR TEENS AND TWENTIES AND MORE

Food Groups	Total Servings Per Day
MILK	4 glasses (8 oz. each)
MEAT (or alternate)	2-3 servings (5 oz. total)
VEGETABLES & FRUITS	
Citrus fruit	1 serving ($1/2$ cup)
Dark green or deep yellow vegetables	1 serving ($1/2$ cup)
Other fruits & vegetables	2 servings ($1/2$ cup each)
BREADS & CEREALS (increase servings as more calories are needed)	4 servings minimum
FATS (margarine & salad oil)	1 to 2 tablespoons
WATER (or other liquid)	8 glasses (includes 4 glasses milk)
SALT (iodized)	Only moderate amount
SUGAR & STUFF	Keep to a minimum!

SUGGESTED MENU PATTERN FOR ATHLETE WORKING OUT IN LATE AFTERNOON

BREAKFAST*	*LUNCH*	*DINNER***
orange juice	cream of vegetable soup	meat (small serving)
cereal	hearty sandwich with	mixed salad greens with
eggs & beef sausage	meat or substitute	oil dressing
toast & jelly	cottage cheese or	small baked potato
milk or cocoa	molded salad	rolls with butter
*(substantial meal — adjust portions to suit calorie needs)	fruit dessert	pudding or
	milk	fruit dessert
		milk
		**(lightest meal)

SUGGESTED MENU PATTERN FOR ATHLETE WORKING OUT IN THE MORNING

BREAKFAST*	*LUNCH***	*DINNER*
orange juice	macaroni & cheese or	cream vegetable soup
cereal or egg	meat casserole	hearty sandwich with
toast & jelly	green salad with	meat or substitute
milk or cocoa	oil dressing	molded fruit or
*(lightest meal)	rolls & butter	vegetable salad
	fruit dessert	fruit dessert
	milk	milk
	**(substantial meal)	

SUGGESTED MENU PATTERN FOR INCREASED MEAL FREQUENCY*

Meal 1: egg or cheese
          whole-grain bread or toast
          milk

Meal 2: fresh fruit or orange juice
            or dried fruit

Meal 3: soup (vegetable or cream type)
          green salad with oil-vinegar dressing

Meal 4: fish or meat or peanut butter sandwich
          fruit or vegetable juice or milk

Meal 5: meat or fish or poultry or cheese
          potato or whole-grain cereal
          leafy green and other vegetables
          milk

Meal 6: fruit
          ice cream (or yogurt)

* Same amount of food as suggested for three meals a day only spaced differently. Some athletes prefer this.

CARBOHYDRATE-PACKING

There are some sports (e.g., any type of rugged, strenuous activity of long duration such as long-distance running or tournament competition) in which performance can be improved by manipulating the diet. For long-duration events, carbohydrates are first choice as an energy supplier, with fats as the supplemental energy source.

Here is a commonly practiced dietary program that many coaches recommend. It is called "carbohydrate-packing." About a week before competition in any endurance event exceeding 30 to 60 minutes, the athlete should exercise to exhaustion the muscles that will be used in competition. He then eats a diet low in carbohydrates but high in proteins and fats for 2 or 3 days. This keeps the glycogen content of the exercising muscles low. Next he switches to a diet high in carbohydrates but with some fats and proteins. The result of this dietary manipulation is what might be called a glycogen overshoot: that is, the body stores more glycogen (the by-product of carbohydrates) than it ordinarily would. Consequently, the athlete can exercise at an intensive rate over longer periods.

Carboydrate-packing is effective but controversial, and for events lasting less than 30 minutes (some coaches even limit carbohydrate-packing to events lasting longer than one and one-half hours) it is probably not necessary. If the athlete slightly increases his fruit and cereal grain intake for a couple of days before an event, it will help to "top off" his glycogen supply without the need for a 5-day routine of carbo-loading. About 3 or 4 hours before the competition the athlete may be permitted to eat what he wants if he thinks it will help him win. Mental state is all-important!

HIGH PROTEIN MENUS*

Breakfast

orange juice
cereal & milk
egg & whole wheat
or enriched toast with margarine,
honey, or jelly
bacon strips
cocoa or skim milk

Breakfast

half of grapefruit
cereal & milk
French toast & syrup
or honey with sausages
cocoa or skim milk

Lunch

chili or hamburger or cheeseburger
relishes (include olives)
vanilla pudding with sliced banana
or fresh banana & glass of skim milk

Lunch

split pea soup with ham
egg salad sandwich with
ripe olives & carrots
milk shake
or glass of skim milk

Dinner

swiss steak
scalloped potatoes
cauliflower with cheese sauce
enriched rolls, margarine, & jelly
custard pie
skim milk

Dinner

fish sticks
rice casserole
dark green lettuce salad
with oil dressing, croutons,
& Parmesan cheese
ice cream sundae

* Adapt size of meal to athlete's needs — increase breakfast, decrease dinner, etc.

HIGH CARBOHYDRATE MENUS*

Breakfast

orange juice or
whole orange
oatmeal with raisins & milk
muffins & jam or jelly
cocoa or milk

Breakfast

orange juice
cereal (granola) & milk
waffles & honey butter
cocoa or milk

Lunch

macaroni salad (lots of
macaroni) with peas
relishes
whole wheat bread & butter
date bars
skim milk

Lunch

potato soup
crackers or crusty bread
relishes
gingerbread or
peach upside-down cake
milk

Dinner

meat loaf
(with bread or oatmeal extender)
baked potato
buttered carrots
cabbage slaw or lettuce with
sweet-sour dressing
apple cake
skim milk

Dinner

spaghetti
(go easy on meat sauce)
baked squash
tossed salad
lots of hot French bread
sugar cookies or
fruit pie
skim milk

* Adapt size of meal to athlete's needs — increase breakfast, decrease dinner, etc.

NUTRITIOUS SNACKS

Proteins

Skim milk & whole milk
Milk shakes
Eggnog & custard
Ice cream
Hard-cooked eggs
Cheese
Peanut butter & nuts
Hamburgers & cheeseburgers
Hot dogs
Pizza, tacos
Chicken livers
Beef jerky

Carbohydrates

Fresh fruits
Dried fruits
Fruit juice
Whole wheat bread
  (in sandwiches & toast)
Vegetable relishes
Fruit bars
Custard & puddings
Grains & seeds
Cereals
Enriched bread & jelly
Sugar cookies

12

Eating Pre-Event, During, and After

CARBOHYDRATES AND LIQUIDS IN—FATS AND PROTEINS OUT (TEMPORARILY)

Several things should be considered in planning pre-event eating. Since energy is one of the prime needs during competition, the intake of carbohydrate foods is important. Choose carbohydrates (such as fruits, vegetables, cereals, and breads) that are easily and quickly digested, those that leave the stomach promptly and are readily absorbed into the bloodstream.

The fat content of pre-event meals should be restricted because fat involves a more complicated digestive process and is slower in its absorption into the cells.

Protein should be avoided in pre-event eating (i.e., during the last few hours), but skim milk is permissible. A meal high in protein will increase the need to urinate; it may produce acidosis, which can result in fatigue. The metabolism of protein into carbohydrate is an energy-consuming process. Thus, it could be detrimental to performance when most energy should go into the athletic activity and not into digesting protein. Protein is *not* essential for energy needs.

Whatever an athlete eats in the last hours before competition can cause trouble. Emotional tension or anxiety may contribute to possible indigestion or a sensation of nausea. If one is prone to such mental states, it is probably better not to eat and to start the competitive event with a hungry feeling.

Eating during strenuous physical exercise forces the body to do an extra load of digestive work. It is not a small matter to push food through 30 feet of tubing. It really is hard physical labor, and the effects on performance are definite and significant. If you can do without eating, you're better off doing so! But if you must eat, eat lightly or try a liquid meal.

LIQUID MEALS

Liquid meals can be the answer to pre-competition eating. The nutrients in liquid meals already are soluble and are quickly digested and absorbed into the body. Liquid meals can be well-balanced in nutrient value, convenient, and economical. They are recommended for consumption from one and one-half to three hours before an athletic event; digestion in the stomach will be completed within that time and there will be little competition between stomach and muscles for the blood supply during the contest.

For athletes who need extra nourishment, a liquid meal can serve as a supplement to the regular light meal preceding the athletic event. For the very nervous individual, a liquid meal may be the most desirable food. It would be a good idea, though, for the athlete to try the liquid meal (same formula as he would be using in competition) prior to his need for it so that he can see whether or not he likes it and how well his stomach tolerates it. However, the very nervous individual might be better off taking a little fruit juice or some hot tea with honey and then eating a complete meal following competition.

Liquid meals should be limited to pre-event use and are suggested nourishment before endurance activities. Liquid meal preparations are helpful in tournaments where an athlete makes several appearances through the day. The period of time between weigh-in and the event (for a wrestler) or between events determines the kind of pre-contest meal. If you use a commercial product, check the label; the formulas vary as to proportions of carbohydrate, protein, and fat. Choose the formula that has the proportion of nutrients you desire, or make your own more economically. (Simple recipes are given in the appendix.)

48 HOURS BEFORE COMPETITION

Avoid	Use
Raw fruits (except oranges, peeled apples, and bananas)	Cooked fruits and vegetables
Raw vegetables (except lettuce)	Fruit and vegetable juices (except prune juice)
Vegetables with seeds	Skim milk
Whole-grain products	Enriched bread, rice, noodles, spaghetti, potatoes, macaroni
Relishes, popcorn, nuts	
Jams, preserves	
Gravy	Roasted and broiled meats
	Cheese
	Eggs (limit of 3 a week)
	Jellies, syrup, and other sweet spreads

24 HOURS BEFORE COMPETITION

Athletes should avoid eating foods that have a tendency to be gas-forming in his or her body. These foods will vary with the athlete, but common offenders include beans of all kinds (except green beans), cabbage, cauliflower, broccoli, and onions.

For all sports activity and particularly out-of-doors events in hot, humid weather, water (and other liquid) consumption is of prime importance. Begin 24 hours before competition to plan consciously for fluid intake—both as to *kind* of liquids and *amounts*.

If the weather is hot on the day of competition, drinking lots of liquids is especially important. The salt content should be neither too little (resulting in the low-sodium syndrome) nor too much (making the athlete thirsty). Good beverages include: skim milk, apple juice, lemonade, orange juice (diluted), tomato juice, clear beef or chicken broth, and bouillon.

For a simple hot-weather drink, add one-fourth teaspoon of salt to one quart of any of the above liquids, or add one teaspoon to six quarts of flavored water. Lemonade or diluted orange juice or tomato juice with a little salt make excellent "exercise" drinks to replace vitamin C. Orange juice and tomato juice also help replace magnesium, which is lost in sweat.

The athlete should get a good night's sleep before competition. Most athletes, even at the college level, function best with eight or nine hours. Each athlete needs to determine how much sleep is best for him. Relieve mental stress as much as possible for best performance; some athletes read, meditate, jog, or even go to a movie the day or evening preceding the "big competition."

MEALS ON DAY OF COMPETITION

Individuals vary in their preference of number and kinds of meals for optimum energy. Each athlete should establish his own pattern according to the sport in which he participates. Many athletes get the jitters before an event; if that happens, it is better to eat lightly. Timing of the meal is also a consideration. A meal should be eaten and digested before time for competition. Size of the meal is a factor; a smaller meal is more easily digested. Eating less but eating more often is desirable.

Foods containing fat should be kept to a minimum in the pre-event meal since fat in any form slows emptying time of the stomach. Liquids consumed before a competition should be low in fat content; hence, skim milk is suggested rather than regular milk.

The athlete may choose a meal that is mostly carbohydrate—on competition day—in preference to the suggested dinner menu three to four hours before or to a liquid meal. A meal of carbohydrates passes out of the stomach within two or three hours.

A light meal consisting of carbohydrates and a small amount of protein (equivalent to that in a glass of skim milk) could be eaten two hours before competition with no adverse effect for most athletes. A simple, predominately carbohydrate meal could consist of toast with a little honey, sugar cookies, banana, and skim milk.

Instead of a regular meal before an event, some athletes prefer a liquid meal. For a person under particular strain and tension, a liquid meal is especially useful since it so easily digested. The liquid may be used alone or it may replace some of the solid foods in a pre-event meal.

Suggested Menu for Meal That May Be Eaten 3-4 Hours Before Competition

1 serving of roasted or broiled lean meat or poultry
1 serving of mashed potato or 1 baked potato
1 serving of cooked vegetable
1 cup skim milk
1 teaspoon margarine, 2 teaspoons jelly with enriched bread
½ cup of cooked fruit or 1 banana
Sugar cookies or plain cake (angel food or sponge)
Extra beverages (1-3 cups) skim milk, bouillon, and fruit juice
Salt food as desired

Suggested Menu for Carbohydrate Meal That May Be Consumed 2 to 3 Hours Before Competition

Orange juice
Baked potato (*or* rice *or* spaghetti and mushroom sauce)
Carrots *or* squash (cooked)
Enriched bread *or* toast with honey *or* jelly
Banana *or* cooked fruit
Sugar cookies *or* angel food cake
Skim *or* low-fat milk

A Liquid Meal That May Be Consumed 2 Hours Before Competition

Non-fat dry milk	½ cup
Skim milk	3 cups
Water	½ cup
Sugar	¼ cup
Flavoring (vanilla)	1 teaspoon

Mix and chill.
1 cup will provide 100 calories.

1½ Hours Before Competition

If the pre-event meal is eaten 3 to 4 hours before the event, another cup of water may be taken 1½ hours before participation. This permits time for elimination of excess fluid before competition.

Within 1 Hour of Competition and Continuing

Quick energy foods do not seem to improve performance in short-term events (including such sports as weight lifting, golf, tennis, and wrestling, unless it is tournament play). Energy for short-term events is already available in the body! Energy supplements do seem to aid performance in endurance events (those of long duration, requiring prolonged effort).

Energy from sugar begins to become available within about 15 minutes of being consumed. Fifty grams of sugar (3 rounded tablespoons, or 200 calories) in a liquid can be taken at 1-hour intervals. For athletes in endurance events this is a valuable supplement to the energy available in body stores. It should be taken in *diluted* solution since fluid in the digestive tract is necessary for absorption. Pure glucose is the most readily available source of energy, but table sugar and honey are digested so quickly that their glucose is available for energy almost as quickly as that from pure glucose.

SUGGESTED MEAL SCHEDULE
ON DAY OF COMPETITION

7:30 A.M.   *Breakfast*

juice
cereal & milk
egg & enriched toast
  (lots of jelly)
milk

10:00 A.M.   *Snack*

granola or
"nuts and bolts"

12:00 P.M.   *Lunch*

tuna sandwich
fruit
milk

4:00 P.M.   *Dinner — Choose from:*

dinner meal (page 149)
carbohydrate meal (page 149)
liquid meal (page 150)

6:30 P.M.   Before 8 P.M. event—
more water!

During Competition

Stored energy is used. Carbohydrate food is burned for energy in the body; it is stored as glycogen in the liver and muscle tissue and as glucose in the body fluid. When more energy is needed, glycogen is released from the liver storehouse and converted to glucose. Training and conditioning improve the ability to use body energy stores. Trained athletes do not become completely exhausted, are able to exercise longer, and use almost all their body carbohydrate reserve.

Water is needed. A primary concern of competing athletes

should be their water intake. When engaged in endurance sports, athletes should drink water during competition. Best performance is achieved by replacing water lost in sweat; otherwise the body becomes dehydrated and suffers fatigue.

After the Competition

Extra salt may be needed when heavy exercise and hot weather cause excessive sweating. During intense physical activity, a loss of two pounds of weight represents a loss of one quart of sweat and a sodium depletion of ½ to 1 gram (¼ to ½ teaspoon). Weight loss thus becomes the guide for water and salt replacement. Bouillon and broth are liquds that take care of both salt depletion and dehydration, and they are often better tolerated than salt tablets. For most athletes, salting food at each meal will take care of sodium requirements.

Fruit juice is good nourishment immediately following competition.

Rest periods after strenuous exercise are especially necessary. The muscles need time to dispose of the waste products and replenish their supply of energy.

Food is not needed by the body at this time for immediate energy. The liver is one storehouse and body fat is another from which the body can draw nutrients for energy, but the athlete may be thinking of food and declare that he or she is "famished!"

Traveling Out of Town

Touring athletes are often on their own when it comes to meals, but advance planning and development of a routine help to make road trips more pleasant. Advance planning could mean that team members bring sack lunches from home, or the coach could make arrangements with a restaurant and order a specific meal for the entire team.

Often, athletic teams will favor "drive-ins" and "quick-serve" establishments. Fortunately, hamburgers, cheeseburgers, fishwiches, and milk shakes are *good foods*. But a word of caution: when eating away from home, choose reputable eating establishments. Food poisoning is especially uncomfortable and inconvenient for competing athletes. How well the athletes fare with their on-the-road eating depends upon their own initiative, their coach's instructions, their budget, and their nutritional knowledge.

13

Less Traditional Eating Practices

THE VEGETARIAN WAY

The term *vegetarian* has several meanings. A strict vegetarian, known also as a "vegan," uses only plant sources for food; he eats *no* animal products. The vegan may get all the nutrients he needs, except vitamin B-12, from plant sources. He will need a supplemental source for B-12.

Another class of vegetarians is known as "lacto-ovo-vegetarians;" they add milk, other dairy products, and eggs to their plant foods. Some vegetarians also eat fish and other sea products.

During the centuries that preceded us, there lived people of many cultures that did not eat meat. Diets of the early Greek athletes, for instance, consisted primarily of fruits, vegetables, and grain products, with very little meat. But during later Greek eras, the meat diet was introduced for athletes as distinctly opposite to the prevailing diet. Since that time,

154

there have been advocates of both types of diets for the athletes in training: one diet consists primarily of high protein meat products; the other is either strictly vegetarian or limited vegetarian.

Vegetarian diets can be adapted to the athlete in an active sports program if foods are selected with knowledge and care. However, some people have little knowledge of how their body works and therefore have no judgment concerning which foods they should select for physical health. There have been some rigidly restricted diets advocated in recent years, and they have been the cause of some real nutrition problems due to lack of certain vitamins and trace minerals.

A major problem with vegetarian diets is in obtaining all of the "essential" amino acids necessary for optimal protein metabolism in the body. Protein quality is dependent upon the amount and availability of the eight "essential" amino acids. They all are contained in protein foods of animal origin. The vegetarian must take special care to include a variety of whole-grain cereals, dried peas, beans, nuts, and a variety of fruits and vegetables in order to get these "essential" amino acids. Grain products are low in lysine, and dried peas and beans are low in methionine; therefore, they are considered to be low-quality proteins. However, when grain products and peas and beans are eaten in the same meal, an adequate balance is provided. Other nutrients such as calcium, iron, and riboflavin also may be in short supply in a strict vegetarian diet.

Most nuts are a valuable source of fat, protein, iron, and B vitamins, but they lack vitamins A, C, and D, and most of them are low in calcium, except almonds. (Vegetarians use almonds as a major source of calcium in their diet.)

Obtaining a sufficient calcium allowance is one of the problems in planning vegetarian meals. Green leafy vegetables are a good source of calcium, but including them and other calcium-rich foods in quantities to substitute for the calcium in milk and other dairy products requires skillful planning. There is little chance of getting too much calcium since the intestine will exercise some control over the amount absorbed. The addition of milk and other dairy products and eggs to the diet (as in the lacto-ovo-vegetarian diet) greatly reduces the possibility of nutritional inadequacies.

There has been very little experimental research done to support or negate the values of a vegetarian diet as a means of increasing physical well-being. The available evidence does not show that a vegetarian diet has either a beneficial or detrimental effect upon physical performance.

Vegetarians are gaining converts to their style of eating. The choice of a vegetarian diet is the athlete's decision, but he or she should be knowledgeable of nutritional principles before embarking upon a complete vegetarian regimen.

FOOD VALUE OF BEANS, CEREALS, SEEDS AND NUTS

Composition per Ounce (28 gram)

	Cal.	Protein (g)	Fat (g)	Carbo-hydrate (g)	Calcium (mg)	Iron (mg)	Thiamine (mg)	Riboflavin (mg)	Niacin (mg)
BEANS									
Navy	95	6	0.4	6.1	30	1.7	0.15	0.04	0.4
Kidney	95	7	0.5	6.1	30	2.2	0.15	0.06	0.6
Soy	110	10	5.0	3.1	57	2.0	0.3	0.09	0.6
Pea (split, dry)	95	7	0.3	5.9	20	1.5	0.22	0.06	0.7
CEREALS									
Corn	105	2.9	1.3	20	3	0.7	0.09	0.03	0.6
Oats	110	3.4	2.1	19	17	1.4	0.1	0.04	0.3
Rice (polished)	100	2.0	0.1	23	1.4	0.3	0.02	0.01	0.3
Wheat (whole)	100	3.3	0.6	20	9	1.0	0.1	0.02	1.4
NUTS									
Almonds	190	6.0	17	3.5	40	1.0	0.1	0.2	1.3
Cashews	170	6.0	13	7	14	1.4	0.2	0.06	0.6
Peanuts	170	8.0	14	5	17	0.7	0.26	0.04	4.8
SEEDS									
Sesame	170	6.0	14	4.6	430	2.8	0.3	0.07	1.4
Sunflower	150	8.0	10	6.5	30	2.0	0.5	0.06	1.7

Figures for this chart are adapted from *The Value of Food* by Patty Fisher and Arnold E. Bender, Oxford University Press (London), 2nd edition, 1975.

ORGANICALLY GROWN FOODS

All foods are organic, but organically grown foods are products of plants grown in soil enriched with humus and compost; chemical fertilizers, chemical pesticides, and herbicides are not used. Organic foods usually are marketed at higher prices than regularly marketed vegetables and fruits, but there is no way of being certain that foods sold or promoted as "organically grown" actually were raised under organic conditions.

There is no federal agency or law that defines and supervises the label "organic" and certifies that such foods fit that description. Legislation for government certification has been introduced, but there is at present no law requiring government inspection of farms claiming to produce organically grown foods. Since organically grown foods in the market are not subject to inspection, the consumer will need to judge whether he is getting the " extra quality" for his money.

No significant difference in nutritional content between regularly and organically grown foods has been reported by the United States Department of Agriculture. *Quantity* and *quality* of food available in our markets have never been better. There is no justification for claiming that "organically grown foods are the only safe source of fruits and vegetables."

The main harm from pesticides, a fear of many people, seems to be the threat to wildlife rather than to humans. One of our major concerns should be that if America's farmers returned to organic farming without benefit of pesticides, herbicides, and chemical fertilizers, there would be a danger that all but about 20 percent of the foods available to us would disappear, and millions of people around the world would starve.

HEALTH FOODS

"Health foods" are as old as mankind. They date from the time when the chief method of healing was to eat something unusual or even repulsive, reasoning that the more distasteful it was, the better the cure.

The health of an individual is the result of many factors, one of which is the food consumed. The body does not require any particular food, but it needs some 50 nutrients in varying amounts from the food supply. Some of these nutrients are required only in trace amounts, others in larger quantities. It is up to us to learn what and how much our body requires.

With each new discovery of much-publicized vitamins and nutrients have come "miracle" pills and potions, "health foods," and some far-out ideas—all of which are dispersed in some health food stores. Much of the faith in "health foods" is developed from the recommendation and encouragement of the "nutrition counselor" behind the cash register. People are eager to believe a promise of wished-for results or cures; but without nutrition knowledge they are victims of many false promises. And many of these victims are athletes, eager to benefit from claims of super strength, super power, and super endurance.

RELYING ON SUPPLEMENTS

Protein Supplements

The quality of protein provided by such foods as meat, fish, poultry, eggs, cheese, and milk make them the best sources of tissue-building material, but remember how exercise and carbohydrates function in muscle building. (See "Energy Requirements For Gaining Muscle—Not Fat" in Chapter 8). The diet of most athletes contains an excessive amount of protein without need of protein supplements.

Since muscular growth takes place slowly and is not dependent on large protein intakes, massive amounts of protein or protein supplements are not required and may actually be a liability, both physically and financially. The digestion and excretion of non-used protein can cause stress on both the liver and the kidneys.

Protein supplements include protein pills and protein

powders made from what may seem to some very unappetizing substances such as powdered liver, beef organs, and yeast; but in addition, such items as skimmed milk powder, egg whites, and soy beans may be included. Read the label to know *what* and *how much* protein is in the formula. Small amounts of fat and carbohydrate often are included.

Sometimes an athlete receives psychological benefit from consuming a supplement alleged to have remarkable powers. Usually, the consumption of protein tablets is the result of smart advertising. Intensive exercise and good food should be sufficient for most athletes in an athletic program. (Note: liquid protein is sold as a diet supplement for weight reduction—see Chapter 22 for further information.)

Vitamin Supplements

Vitamins present in fruits and vegetables, as well as milk, meats, and cereals eaten regularly, enable an athlete to satisfy his daily vitamin needs, and *no vitamin tablets are necessary.* There is no evidence that large supplements of vitamins above the recommended daily allowance improve athletic performance.

Mineral Supplements

A normal, well-balanced diet provides a sufficient supply of the minerals necessary for body processes in athletic competition. Some athletes, not realizing the rich sources of minerals in a variety of foods, are taking tablets containing calcium, phosphorous, magnesium, iron, and iodine in hopes of increasing performance. That is not always necessary. The only mineral supplement that perhaps is needed is iron and that only under certain conditions, which are discussed on the following pages.

Iron Supplements

Iron supplements are needed only in the case of an indicated iron deficiency. An iron deficiency usually is created simply by not eating enough food to allow the body to absorb sufficient iron, by not eating good iron-rich foods (liver, eggs, green leafy vegetables, whole-grain and enriched cereals), by sudden growth, by blood donation, or, in the case of females, by unusual amounts lost through menstruation.

The body stores approximately 1,000 mg (1 gm) of iron: 30 percent is stored in the liver; 30 percent in the bone marrow; and the rest in the spleen and muscles. A reserve of 1,000 mg would last a male adult 1,000 days and would last an adult female about 500 days. Iron-rich foods help build up a reserve of iron in the body. Only when the body's reserves of iron have been depleted will there be any evidence of iron-deficiency symptoms.

Since the body has no mechanism for excreting iron, the iron content of the body, both functioning iron and storage iron, is regulated through controlled absorption. Thus, iron seems to be absorbed in the body in response to a need. (This is in contrast to vitamin C, which is water soluble, and amounts not needed by the body are simply excreted in the urine.) With iron, the body controls the amount it stores by simply not absorbing extra amounts. A person with normal hemoglobin levels absorbs from 2 to 10 percent of dietary iron while a person with low hemoglobin levels and probably high demands for iron may absorb as much as 60 percent of dietary iron.

The presence of a reducing substance such as an acid is believed to enhance iron absorption. Organic acids in foods, such as ascorbic acid (vitamin C) found in citrus fruits, enhance iron absorption. The hydrochloric acid secreted in the stomach keeps iron in a readily available reduced form (ferrous iron) for absorption. Amino acids, especially cysteine, increase the proportion of dietary iron absorbed. When meal planning, consider foods that work together for best iron absorption.

The body is extremely efficient in conserving iron and in a very miserly way retains or salvages any iron that results from the breakdown of iron-containing substances. For example, red blood cells have a functioning life of about four months. As these cells die, they are removed from the bloodstream by cells of the liver, bone marrow, and spleen. In the spleen the iron and amino acids of the hemoglobin molecule are removed. The iron is stored in the liver and spleen, or it is returned to the bone marrow, where it is incorporated into new hemoglobin molecules. By this mechanism, iron is conserved carefully and reused in the body.

Iron is present in every cell. The loss of hair, skin, and fingernails represent a daily loss of iron. A small number of red blood cells, containing less than 0.1 mg of iron, appear in the urine; perspiration also is believed to contain some iron. Losses can vary from 0.2 to 1 mg per day from the various above-listed sources. These losses are the only ones that adult males must replace. Iron deficiency in males in the United States is seldom due to nutritional causes.

In addition, women must replace iron lost in menstruation. The average iron loss of 1.2 mg a day for menstruating women can be recovered with an average diet, but normal diets are inadequate for women with 1.5 mg a day iron loss or the more unusual loss of 2 mg a day in heavy menstruation.

For athletes donating blood, iron replacement should be an important consideration since iron in our bodies is used to manufacture hemoglobin, a protein of the red blood cells, which circulates in the blood. The amount of oxygen the blood can carry to the muscles is dependent on the amount of hemoglobin in the blood. When the body is deficient in iron, and, therefore, hemoglobin, body tissues fail to receive their quotas of oxygen.

A loss of 1 pint of blood represents a loss of 250 mg of iron that must be replaced. The volume of blood and the number of red cells will return to normal rather quickly, but the return of hemoglobin to previous levels can occur only at the expense of storage iron. Even with the increased rate of iron absorption that occurs after blood donation, it takes about 50 days to restore normal hemoglobin levels. This period can be reduced to about 35 days if iron supplements and ascorbic acid tablets are taken. Ascorbic acid tablets (vitamin C) influence the increased rate of absorption of iron. One can see the wisdom of limiting blood donations to 4 to 6 pints per year, especially for women who are menstruating regularly.

Since the body is extremely efficient in conserving iron supplies, simple iron deficiencies usually occur only during the growth period or when intake fails to meet needs after loss of blood.

All endurance athletes should be concerned with building up and maintaining a high proportion of hemoglobin in their blood. An athlete deficient in iron is listless and easily exhausted; he also suffers from loss of appetite and may be retarded in growth and more susceptible to disease. An athlete who experiences any of these symptoms would be wise to consult his doctor for a blood test. If iron deficiency is indicated, iron-rich foods can be added to the diet. If iron supplements are also needed, the doctor will so advise.

FASTING

To fast is to abstain from food. Fasting is not damaging to a healthy individual, but an athlete cannot expect to compete effectively if he is deprived of energy sources for extended periods during his training. There is no evidence to suggest that periodic fasting provides any competitive advantage, but some marathon runners feel that fasting is the best possible way to give their body a "change-of-pace," to purge it of unnecessary materials, and to feel a "oneness" with nature.

Some runners even point out that it is best to fast beginning the day before the event because the body does not run on what it consumes just before the event but on the reserves it has built up earlier. Months (and years) of long training help the athlete to use these reserves of energy efficiently. This energy is in the form of glycogen, which is chiefly stored in the liver and some in muscle tissue. Digestion processes shortly before or during a race waste energy.

Short periods of fasting (up to three days) with free access to water or extended periods of fasting (three to seven days) with a low-calorie, high-quality protein intake, such as three glasses of skim milk per day and a multiple vitamin supplement every other day, probably would be a safe recommendation for a healthy mature athlete. Fasting, as practiced by many adults, may have its place among devoted followers, but athletes *still in their growing years* should be counseled to refrain from extensive fasting periods.

The cells of the body, except for erythrocytes (red blood cells formed in the bone marrow) and those of the central nervous system, can utilize fatty acids directly as a source of energy. Carbohydrate is the energy normally used by the nervous system; only after a period of adaptation to total starvation can the brain utilize ketone bodies, which are formed from fatty acids and amino acids.

The principle that before competition as little as possible should be eaten remains a good practice.

THE BREAD DIET—AND A PLEA FOR EATING MORE BREAD

One of the latest diets to make the headlines is fittingly, but unglamorously, named the "bread diet." Interest and enthusiasm for such a diet may have been stimulated by the report early in 1977 from the United States Senate Select Committee on Nutrition and Human Needs. The report suggested dietary changes and recommended changes in food selection and preparation.

One particularly important suggested dietary change was an increase in carbohydrate consumption to about two-thirds of the daily caloric intake. For one consuming 2,000 calories, this could mean about 1,300 calories would be from carbohydrate foods.

In the early part of this century, almost 40 percent of our calories was from carbohydrates—specifically vegetables and fruits, and a very important share was from grain products. (Our ancestors ate hearty breads and hot cereals.) Today we are eating much less whole or cracked grain breads and cereals, fresh vegetables, and fruits, and are eating more foods containing flour, fat, and sugar.

Another reason the Senate Select Committee suggested sweeping changes in our eating habits is that scientists report there is reason to believe that diets high in carbohydrates (vegetables, fruits and grain products—in their natural state— without loss of nutrients due to commercial processing), reduce the risk of developing heart disease, diabetes, bowel cancer, and other diseases of the intestines.

Bread was once regarded as the "staff of life" in most families. Today, many people plan their meals around *not* bread, but hamburger. Since hamburger, or any other red meat, may contain large amounts of fat, the Senate Committee suggests we re-think what kinds of foods containing proteins, fats, and carbohydrates that we include in our daily eating. One way to cut down on fat consumption is to obtain more of our protein requirements from grain and vegetable sources, also fish and poultry. Our bodies need 20 amino acids in the right proportion to produce protein; meat, fish, poultry, and egg contain all of them. Grain and vegetable sources do not contain all 20 and are therefore called incomplete proteins, but by careful planning, and by combining wheat products with other grains and with dairy products, incomplete proteins can become complete proteins. Also, we can get *more* protein from bread by eating it with cheese or a glass of milk.

The Senate Committee notes that bread consumption has been declining and suggests that one reason may be that bread has been viewed *incorrectly* as fattening, and therefore as a "no-no" food. One can hardly call bread a "high-fat food," most breads contain less than 1 gram of fat per slice. It is not the bread, but the butter or margarine spread on the slice of bread that adds the fat, and the jam on top of that that makes the extra calories which the dieter cannot afford.

Adopting the bread diet can be the beginning of a whole new lifetime of eating habits for the athlete and nonathlete alike. The bread diet can be a continuing source of energy and well-being, and can include more carbohydrates (vegetables, fruits, and cereal grains) and less of saturated animal fat, refined sugar, and salt.

Choose bread carefully and read the labels for contents. Some people prefer to make their own. A slice of bread (about 1 ounce per slice) will contain 60 to 80 calories. Eat six slices of bread each day. For variety, you can choose from a wide assortment of breads—such as cracked wheat, pumpernickel, rye, sprouted wheat, white enriched or whole wheat, gluten, oatmeal, etc. Vary your sandwich selections to add variety and good nutritional balance.

Do plan your meals ahead—consider what you are eating for the entire day. Food eaten at one meal should supplement what is eaten at the other meals. By planning, one knows exactly what the body has to operate on.

Bread Diet As a Reducing Diet

The bread diet, besides being an introduction to the concept of increasing one's consumption of whole grain carbohydrates and decreasing the consumption of fats and highly refined carbohydrates, can serve as a weight reduction diet. Bizarre weight reduction diets usually do not provide adequate weight control because of their radical departure from the normal daily diet, but with minor calorie adjustments, the bread diet can become a healthy way of eating and provide for weight reduction or weight maintenance.

On the bread diet, if one is diligent in keeping total calories to around 1,200 a day, one can lose up to two or three pounds, or if one is very heavy, up to four pounds a week. If the dieting is combined with an exercise program, a weight reduction effort can be very successful. The following suggested daily menus can help the dieter stay within the 1,200 calorie limit.

Breakfast—about 240 calories.

Breakfast menu is basically the same every day—two slices of bread with a special spread. (To make the spread, whirl one

8 oz. container of low-fat cottage cheese in a blender with ½ cup of plain yogurt. Keep the spread in a plastic container in the refrigerator. This is enough to last one week. You can flavor it with a little fruit, cinnamon or vanilla.) Drink a glass (6 oz.) of skim milk with your breakfast each morning.

Lunch—about 460 calories.

You should eat your two slices of bread as a sandwich for lunch each day. Choose from a variety of breads. For the filling, you can choose 3 oz. skinless, boneless chicken or turkey; 3 oz. tuna—packed in water; 2 oz. low-fat cheese; or one egg—twice a week. You can use diet margarine, salad dressing, and always include lettuce and tomato. Use celery, carrot slices, or other vegetables to give extra crunch and nutrient value. Drink one glass (6 oz.)' of skim milk, and include a fruit for dessert.

Dinner—about 500 calories.

Each night you should have the following:

1) One 4 oz. serving of broiled or baked fish or poultry. Choose a low-fat fish like sole, flounder, halibut, haddock, ocean perch, cod, tuna (water packed), skinless chicken or turkey.

2) Two servings of different colored vegetables such as carrots and green beans. Include potatoes at least twice a week as one of the vegetables (boil or bake them). Mixed salad as one of the vegetables is also acceptable—with vinegar and oil or yogurt dressing.

3) Two slices of bread or two dinner size rolls. Choose French or Italian or any other bread. Limit spread to 1 teaspoon of margarine.

4) One serving of fruit for dessert.

For weight reduction, do keep your calorie intake to 1,200 (or less) a day. After you have been on the diet for a few days, you can substitute 2/3 cup of rice (try brown rice), or 1 cup pasta in place of your bread at dinner; or 1 serving of whole grain cereal with skim milk can be substituted for bread at breakfast.

REFERENCES FOR FURTHER READING

Books

Howe, P.S., *Basic Nutrition in Health and Diseases*. Philadelphia: W.B. Saunders, 6th ed. 1976.

Hueneman, R.L., M.C. Hampton, A.B. Behnke, L.R. Shapiro, and B.W. Mitchell. *Teenage Nutrition and Physique*. Springfield, Illinois: Charles C. Thomas, 1974.

Lappe, F.M. *Diet for a Small Planet*. Rev. ed. New York: Ballantine Books, 1975.

Mayer, Jean. *Overweight: Causes, Cost, and Control*. Englewood Cliffs, New Jersey: Prentice-Hall, 1968.

White, P.L., and N. Selvey. *Let's Talk About Food*. Chicago: Follett, 1975.

Periodicals

Astrand, P. "Something Old and Something New—Very New (Carbohydrate Packing)," *Nutrition Today*, 3(2): 9-11 (June 1968).

Bergstrom, J., and E. Heltman. "Nutrition for Maximal Sports Performance," *J.A.M.A*, 221:999-1006 (1972).

Dwyer, J.T., D. Mayer. K. Dowd, R.F. Kandel, and J. Mayer "The New Vegetarians: The Natural High?" (*J. Am. Dietet. A.*, 65:529 (1974).

Harland, B.F., and M. Peterson. "Nutritional Status of Lacto-ovo-vegetarian Trappist Monks," *J. Am. Dietet. A.*, 72:259 (March 1978).

Huse, D.M., and R.A. Nelson. "Basic, Balanced Diet Meets Requirement of Athlete," *The Phy. and Sportsmed.*, 5:53-56 (January 1977).

McBean, L.D., and E.W. Speckman "Food Faddism: A Challenge to Nutritionists and Dietitians, *Am. J. Clin. Nutr.*, 27:1071 (October 1974).

"Nutritional Aspects of Vegetarianism, Health Foods, and Fad Diets," *Nutrition Reviews*, 35:153-57 (June 1977).

Paul, Dr. William. "Crash Diets and Wrestling," *Journal of the National Athletic Trainers Association* (Winter 1966).

Wong, N. P., D. E. LaCroix, and J. A. Alford. "Mineral Content of Dairy Products—Milk and Milk Products," *J. Am. Dietet. A.,* 72:288 (1978).

Wurtman, J., W. Sammons, B. Brazelton, F. Crawford, and M. Winick. "Four-part Nutrition Plan for Good Health," *Parents,* 53:37-39 (March 1978).

part 4

Problems in Performance

14
Body Fluid

Body fluid, consisting of water and dissolved minerals, is an electrically charged fluid that serves as a medium for important life functions such as the movement of nutrients and transfer of oxygen and other materials in the tissues. The body fluid contains several minerals that serve as ions for electrolytes, which means that they are elements that have electrical charges that enable them to react with other minerals in the body fluid. (See "Magnesium," "Potassium," and "Sodium" in Chapter 6.) These electrolytes partially control the chemical balance of the body, and they function best in a slightly alkaline fluid.

The minerals that must be supplied by our diet, and which have such important functions in the body fluid, include sodium, potassium, calcium, and magnesium. Sodium and potassium are in the highest concentration in body fluid. Sodium is concentrated predominantly in the *extracellular* fluid (outside of body cells). Potassium is concentrated in the *intracellular* fluid (within body cells). The composition of the fluids within and outside the cells is quite different. The extracellular fluid contains a large amount of sodium and chlorine and is equivalent to a 0.9 percent solution of common salt (sodium chloride). Small amounts of potassium, calcium, magnesium, phosophorous, and sulfur also are present. In addition to these inorganic salts, the extracellular fluid contains dissolved carbon dioxide, protein, a small amount of organic acids, and other organic compounds.

The intracellular fluid is high in potassium and phosphorus. It also contains more magnesium, sulfur, and protein than does the extracellular fluid but less carbon dioxide and much less sodium.

The body fluid is distributed as follows: approximately 35 percent *within* cells as intracellular fluid; approximately 25 percent *between* cells as extracellular fluid; and the remainder (approximately 40 percent) in the circulating blood.

The distribution of water in the blood and in the intracellular and extracellular fluid is determined by the delicate balance of mineral salt concentration and amount of water in the body. If there is a marked decrease in body-water consumption or a marked increase in salt consumption, this will affect the sweat-cooling process. The body's functions will be greatly affected because of decreasing water in the intracellular area and increasing water by osmotic pressure effects in the extracellular. The major function of electrolytes is to control and maintain the correct rate of fluid exchange within the various fluid compartments of the body.

For best performance, water should be available for intracellular functions and not be retained between cells in the extracellular compartments. That can best be done by limiting intake of salt and replacing lost water with plain water. This hastens replenishment of body fluid to the intracellular spaces, where it is most needed.

Body fluid is not excess weight, and athletes should realize that if this distribution of body fluid so critically balanced within and outside the cell walls is disturbed by extreme measures when trying to lose weight (for example, by limiting the drinking of water), it can result in serious complications.

If there is rapid or prolonged dehydration, the electrolyte balance is upset, leading to decrease of mental alertness, sluggishness, weakness, lack of muscular coordination, neuralgic disturbances, and stress on the cardiovascular system.

Plan to replenish electrolytes lost through sweat by eating mineral-rich vegetables and fruits. Tomato and orange juice, green leafy vegetables, whole-grain cereals, fish, meat, nuts, and milk are all good sources for electrolyte replacements (see chart for listing of minerals).

Electrolyte	Food Source*
Calcium	Cheeses (Cheddar) Milk and milk products Vegetables (leafy, dark green) Fish (canned, soft bones)
Chlorine	Table salt (NaCl)
Magnesium	Breads (whole wheat) Cereals (wheat bran and germ) Legumes (beans, peas, peanuts) Nuts Vegetables (leafy) Cocoa
Potassium	Lean meats (including hamburger) Chicken Fruits (bananas, oranges, apples, cantaloupe, dates) Tomato juice Vegetables (leafy dark green) Carrots (raw) Potatoes (french fries) Potato chips (salted)
Phosphorus	Meats (especially organ meats) Fish Poultry Eggs Milk and Cheese Grains Nuts Seeds Fruits (dried)

Electrolyte	Food Source*
Sodium	Cheeses (Cheddar)
	Eggs
	Rice
	Pickle (dill)
	Potato chips (salted)
	Popcorn (with oil and salt)
	Table salt (NaCl)
Sulfur	Cabbage
	Eggs
	Onions

*"Nutritive Value of Foods", Home and Garden Bulletin No. 72, United States Department of Agriculture, revised January, 1971; also adapted from NUTRITION AND PHYSICAL FITNESS, -Bogert, Briggs and Calloway, 9th Edition, 1973.

EXERCISE DRINKS

An "exercise" drink is a beverage designed to serve as a thirst-satisfying means of replacing minerals and water lost in perspiration. It is sometimes referred to as an electrolyte, isotonic, or action drink.

Exercise drinks are mostly water, but they do vary in their formulas. They have three things in common: they replace lost fluid with water, they replace lost glycogen with sugar, and they replace lost electrolyte ions, usually sodium but sometimes potassium or one of the other electrolyte ions. Chief electrolyte ions present in the body are the positively charged sodium, potassium, calcium, magnesium, phosphorus, and sulfur ions and negatively charged chlorine.

Since athletes in various sports lose different minerals in varying proportions through sweat, one kind of exercise drink does not work most efficiently for all. Individuals and coaches will need to decide what ingredients and what proportions are important for their sport and for the people involved. Since sweat contains approximately one-fourth teaspoon of salt per quart (this will vary a little with different athletes), a good exercise drink includes the same proportions of salt to water. Sweeteners also go into the exercise drink for palatability and caloric replacement. By including both quick-acting and slower-acting sugars such as glucose and sucrose, one can have sweetness as well as an immediate and a slightly delayed release of energy to the bloodstream. However, if too sweet, such a sugar solution will draw fluid from the body cells into the stomach, which may cause cramps.

Because vitamin C is lost in sweat (it is vital to the metabolism of glucose), it is important to include it in an exercise drink.

It takes 30 minutes (or more) to get the full effect from a water-mineral-glucose drink. So if you are depending on benefits from an exercise drink during your performance, time your drink accordingly.

Check formulas of exercise drinks for their mineral content. Potassium has been isolated as one of three important minerals lost during athletic competition (sodium and magnesium are the other two). Increased potassium excretion with increased salt intake also is observed in hot climates. However, potassium is so widely distributed in foods of both plant and animal origin that it is easy to get sufficient amounts to satisfy daily requirements. In fact, the ingestion of potassium is so great that nearly all potassium ingested in the average diet is quite promptly excreted in the urine (with a small amount retained for use in normal cell replacement and the repair of body tissue). Because of our high intake of potassium-carrying foods, it is not necessary to select an electrolyte drink especially for its potassium content.

Dr. Donald L.Cooper, Director of Oklahoma State University Student Hospital and Clinic and researcher, has concluded that the main mineral drain in marathon running is magnesium. He suggests that the endurance athlete should be concerned with consuming foods and liquids containing magnesium rather than gobbling salt tablets or drinking commercial salt-replacement solutions. (See "Magnesium" in Chapter 6 for suggestions of magnesium-rich foods.)

Because phosphorus is vital to the liberation of energy—it helps control the rate at which energy is released in the body—and also because phosphorus can regulate the acid content of the blood, some coaches and trainers recommend that their athletes consume special "phosphate drinks" three to four hours prior to competition to improve performance. Although some people have attributed enhanced performance to these drinks, there is no scientific evidence in support of this practice.

It should be stated further that there have been no studies that support claims for improved performance resulting from the use of any of the exercise drinks. Our best advice is to drink lots of water, and if you must buy a so-called "exercise" or "electrolyte" drink know what you are getting besides expensive water.

The following homemade electrolyte drinks have minerals and/or vitamins in addition to the water content: skim milk has both sodium and potassium (also calcium); orange juice contains magnesium and is high in potassium and vitamin C but lacks sodium; tomato juice is high in potassium and also has vitamin C; and lemonade has potassium. Formulas for other suggested exercise drinks are included in the appendix.

THE SALT OF THE EARTH

In the past it was advocated that the athlete take salt tablets and do heavy salting of food, but now we are realizing that salt in large amounts is not as essential a supplement to the athlete's diet as once believed. In fact, the average American's diet is unnaturally high in salt. Because everything we eat and drink contains some salt, the body's need can be met from natural sources—without turning to the salt shaker.

Salt tablets taken alone without adequate fluids can do more harm than good. Often, it is the lack of an adequate supply of water nearby that is the problem. The salt tablets are convenient and easy to take; in fact, they are so easy to take that an athlete often decides that if two are good, why not take four. But the individual may decide that it is too much trouble to get the necessary water to accompany the tablets, so the salt is consumed without sufficient liquid. As a precaution, water should be consumed, in adequate quantity, before the salt tablet.

Another current concern about salt tablets is that they too often are taken just prior to an activity. Because they are slow in dissolving, the salt won't be dissolved until two or three hours after ingesting, when the fluid in the cells may be at a lower level due to sweating. Having a salt tablet at breakfast would be a better practice. Perhaps still better would be eliminating the salt tablet and lightly salting the food instead—if a little extra salt is needed.

It is now thought that high salt intake accelerates sweating, and in the process other essential electrolytes (such as potassium, calcium, and magnesium) are lost along with the sodium chloride—giving the athlete a "washed-out" feeling.

The body has highly effective mechanisms for regulating its elimination of salt. The hormone aldosterone regulates the amount of sodium excreted in the urine. Also, under the influence of this hormone, the sweat glands participate in the control by reducing the concentration of salt in sweat when water losses through sweating are high.

Conditioned runners have discovered that their sweat is more dilute. A conditioned body adapts to heat, the sweat glands work more efficiently, and the body seems to conserve electrolytes.

If the body has become dependent on large salt doses, we need to be weaned away carefully. The best time to cut down on salt is during the cool-weather months. Then, when summer arrives the athlete will be better adjusted to a reduced salt intake, and he can judge how well he copes with heat and humidity.

Salt and water are both important to an athlete, and remember—salt a little but water a lot!

THINK WATER

And now we'll say it again—think water! At least eight glasses of liquid a day. Since water is considered so important to the health of the athlete, it is dealt with separately in Chapter 1.

It is mandatory for an athlete to realize the importance of his water intake. No one has been known to starve during an athletic event (most athletes are over-fed), but some participants have been permanently disabled or have died for lack of sufficient water.

Remember, thirst is a warning signal that the body needs water. It should be responded to promptly. The temperature of the water drunk is unimportant, but drinking it is.

A source of clean water should be conveniently located for the athletes. Many won't bother to walk a mile for a drink of water. Disposable cups are helpful; a common dipper might foster spread of undesirable microorganisms.

It is desirable that athletes keep a container of water handy in the refrigerator at home as a reminder to drink more water early and late each day. Cool or cold water is more inviting than lukewarm. You don't need to worry about drinking too much water because the kidneys will unload the excess in a matter of a few hours.

An athlete should check his or her weight at a regular time each day—any loss is probably a water loss. Checking weight is the most accurate determinant of your water need.

Think water! Drink water! Take at least eight glasses of liquid a day!

15
Problems to Avoid

OVERHEATING

Since prevention is the most important way to deal with overheating, sun stroke, or heat exhaustion, a few suggestions will be given in hopes that they will be of particular benefit to athletes who are exposed to such dangers.

In many areas fall football practice begins during hot, sometimes humid, sticky weather, and the athletes are not yet acclimatized. The weather can be so humid that perspiration will not even permit surface cooling. If temperature is high and humidity low, sweat will evaporate, but if temperature is high and humidity is high also, effective evaporation will not be possible.

In hot, humid weather one should avoid practice sessions during the warmest part of the day—especially at the beginning of the school year when the athlete is not conditioned. Practice sessions in the morning and evening are preferable in order to avoid the heat.

Football uniforms and protective gear pretty well cover the

body, preventing necessary sweating that allows the body to cool. During exercise periods in especially hot weather, wear loose, porous clothing if possible—preferably of a light color.

Know the signs of overheating, heat exhaustion, and heat stroke as well as the treatment for each. Be aware of dizziness, extreme fatigue, muscle cramps, or even coordination problems, which might signify heat difficulties. Report them immediately to your coach. Talk with your coaching staff about emergency procedures in case of illness.

If the water supply is inadequate or inconvenient, the athlete will not bother to drink. The longer drinking is delayed, the more intense the heat in the body. Since the feeling of thirst lags behind the need for water, water breaks at regular intervals are important. Plain water (without sugar) is absorbed into the body cells fastest.

Record weights each evening (at a regular time), especially during hot weather, as a guide to replenishing liquid. Plan to replenish at least a pint of fluid for each pound lost—that amount is minimum.

To help avoid overheating problems, *drink plenty of good water* and wear loose, lightweight clothing.

Heat Exhaustion

Symptoms: The face is pale (ashen), perspiration is profuse, and the entire body may be clammy. The pulse is weak, breathing shallow and the person usually feels extremely weak. Sometimes a brief period of unconsciousness or fainting will ensue. Nausea, vomiting, dizziness, and unsteadiness are almost always present. Temperature is approximately normal.

Treatment: The person should lie down—with head at the same level as the rest of the body or slightly lower—in a well-ventilated, airy place. He should be lightly covered and given a half-teaspoon of salt in about half a glass of water, continuing this treatment until he has consumed a glass or more of water. Warm coffee or tea may be drunk. If symptoms continue, a doctor should be called. It is believed that the value of salt has been overemphasized and that the intake of liquids is of vital importance.

Heat Cramps: Symptoms and Treatment

Heat cramps are extremely painful and usually affect the muscles in the arms and legs or abdominal muscles. Heat cramps may be accompanied by symptoms of heat exhaustion, and the treatment is the same as for heat exhaustion. Firm hand pressure on the affected area sometimes gives relief.

Sunstroke

Symptoms: The individual's face is flushed, and the skin is hot and dry. The pulse is rapid, and the body temperature can be 107° or higher. The patient ordinarily feels dizziness and headache, dryness of the mouth and skin, and nausea. Unconsciousness can follow rapidly, and about one-fourth of all serious cases end fatally. Prompt action is important. Although the body usually is relaxed, convulsions sometimes occur.

Treatment: The person should be placed on his back, with head slightly elevated, in a cool place and clothes removed. Wet cloths or ice bags should be applied to cool the head. Cool the body by wrapping the patient in a sheet or cloth and pouring on small amounts of cold water. The body should not be cooled too rapidly. Arms and legs should be massaged, through the sheet, in the direction of the heart to aid circulation. Another way to cool the body is by immersion in cool water for about 20 minutes. Ice bags also may be used. The cooling treatment and massage should continue until the skin no longer appears hot and flushed. No stimulants should be given, but when conscious, the person may have cool drinks. A doctor should be called as soon as possible.

Heatstroke: Symptoms and Treatment

The signs to watch for in heatstroke are dizziness, drowsiness, and fast breathing. When the attack occurs, it is essential to transfer the victim at once to a cool place, and then keep him flat on his back and absolutely quiet. Sponging with cool water will help to control the temperature, and the circulation may be stimulated with coffee or other stimulants. Some authorities advise that the victim of heatstroke be placed on a cot covered with a rubber sheet; his entire body then is rubbed with ice until the temperature drops to 102° degrees. At that point, the cold treatment is terminated and the patient covered with blankets. If breathing stops, it is necessary to administer artificial respiration at once.

KETOSIS (OR ACIDOSIS)

Ketosis is a condition that occurs in the body when fatty acids are not completely metabolized and intermediary products called *ketones* accumulate in the bloodstream.

A healthy individual, consuming a normal well-balanced diet, is not likely to develop ketosis, but athletes most susceptible to a ketosis condition are young wrestlers who are determined to reduce their weight by a complete starvation-crash-diet scheme.

Carbohydrate is an important source of energy for muscle contraction, but the body's stores are limited to small amounts of glycogen in muscles and liver. As the carbohydrate stores are used during fasting, tissue protein is metabolized to provide just enough carbohydrate to maintain brain function. But the carbohydrate stores are then depleted and the body shifts to using fat as its major source of energy. This presents a problem because carbohydrate is needed for the most efficient utilization of fat. When carbohydrate is scarce, fat is not completely oxidized and intermediary substances called keto acids or ketones are formed. Thus, in fasting, the lack of carbohydrate and the overuse of fat lead to ketosis.

Ketones accumulate in the body, and then when they are excreted in the urine, they carry with them essential minerals, which results in a reduction of the slightly alkaline reserve of the blood and a condition of acidosis.

Another consequence of ketosis is a reduced uptake of carbohydrate into the muscles with resultant reduction in available carbohydrate energy, which leads to a feeling of fatigue.

A ketosis condition also results in a loss of potassium, which follows cellular breakdown. Potassium is one of the minerals essential to efficient muscle function.

CARBOHYDRATE FOODS*

Food	Amount (1 cup = 8 ounces)	Carbohydrates (grams)
Pudding (choc.)	1 cup	67
Sherbet	1 cup	59
Beans (baked with pork and molasses)	1 cup	54
Pea soup (split)	1 cup	52
Chicken pot pie	4½" diam.	42
Macaroni and cheese	1 cup	40
Spaghetti with meat balls and tomato sauce	1 cup	39
Sweet potato (baked)	1 medium	36
Dates (pitted)	¼ cup	33
Squash (winter-baked)	1 cup	32
Raisins	¼ cup	32
Pizza (sausage)	⅙ of 14" (diameter)	30
Chili (with beans)	1 cup	30
Watermelon	1 wedge (4x8")	27
Cocoa	1 cup	27
Apricots (dried)	10 halves	25
Potato (white, baked)	1 medium	21
Corn (canned)	½ cup	20
Orange	1 medium	16
Bread (whole wheat)	1 slice	14
Grapefruit	½ medium	12
Milk (skim)	1 cup	12
Tomato juice	1 glass (6 oz)	8

*Adapted from figures in "Nutritive Value of Foods", Home and Garden Bulletin No. 72, United States Department of Agriculture, revised, January, 1971.

An athlete who is trying to diet should include a minimum of 70 grams of carbohydrates a day in order to avoid ketosis (e.g., 1 cup of skim milk or 1 slice of bread = 12 grams of carbohydrate).

While some may view with delight the prospect of rapid weight loss on a carbohydrate-free diet, the physiological changes which accompany this condition are certainly undesirable and potentially hazardous.

The wrestlers who count on complete carbohydrate-free crash dieting can expect to experience early fatigue and a lack of mental alertness. They are the wrestlers who may look good for the first two or three minutes, but will begin to wilt and are outmaneuvered during the second period and may be pinned in the third period.

HYPOGLYCEMIA

Hypoglycemia (low blood sugar) is a "disease" which more and more people claim to have symptoms for, but the healthly, normal athlete should have no trouble with hypoglycemia.

Energy is supplied to the cells in the form of glucose which circulates in the blood and is popularly known as blood sugar. The body has delicate controls over the amount of glucose circulating in the blood. We may envision that there is a large supply of blood sugar, but actually only about 1/10 of 1 percent of the blood is blood sugar. This is a source of ready fuel for our cells.

A certain amount of glucose is stored in muscle tissue and liver in the form of glycogen. As the muscle uses up its glycogen for energy it draws on the blood sugar. The hormone insulin is needed to move glucose from the blood into the cells. This process lowers the blood sugar and stimulates the secretion of adrenalin and glucagon. These hormones cause the liver to release glucose from its stored glycogen and restore the blood sugar level to normal. Thus, it is the balance between these hormones that maintains the circulating glucose within narrow limits. If insufficient insulin is produced to move the blood sugar into the cells, the blood sugar rises to an abnormally high level and the condition is knows as *hyperglycemia*. Some of the excess sugar may be excreted in the urine. On the other hand, if too much insulin is produced, or if glucose fails to mobilize the liver glycogen, the blood sugar falls to an abnormally low level, a condition known as *hypoglycemia*.

In a fasting person the blood sugar stays at a constant level—well within the normal range. Only after a meal does it rise, thereby calling for an outpouring of insulin. Many athletes take extra sugar, dextrose, or honey before a contest. This intake of sugar provides, in a very short time, a rise in the blood sugar level. It is difficult for the athlete to know whether he or she really needs this added sugar, or if exercise is needed to trigger the release of energy he already has stored in his body. Blood sugar needs to get into the muscle cells in order to be of benefit in exercise.

Moderate exercise doesn't bring about hypoglycemia. Hypoglycemia may occur in intense, exhausting exercise, in severe carbohydrate depletion, in overfunctioning of insulin, or in undersecretion of glucagon.

If the athlete feels unusually tired, sluggish, and irritable during or after workouts, it could be a sign of hormone imbalance and it would be wise to ask a doctor to do a glucose tolerance test.

Not all weariness is due to a hypoglycemic state. Accumulation of lactic acid is greater in the untrained athlete than the trained and is due to lack of oxygen when glucose is metabolized. Lactic acid accumulation results in weariness and pain, but after a rest period, when sufficient oxygen is present, lactic acid is converted back to pyruvic acid and is used for energy.

CHOLESTEROL

Athletes hear about *cholesterol*, saturated, and polyunsaturated fats and may wonder what difference all these fats make to them. Ever since cholesterol, a waxy, fatlike material was found in deposits within the inner lining of blood vessels, much concern has been expressed about fats and even about the popular breakfast foods—eggs and bacon, which are common food sources of cholesterol. The effects of the fatty deposits within the blood vessels are to narrow the channel and eventually restrict the flow of blood from the heart and lungs. This condition, called atherosclerosis can lead to heart problems.

The amount of fatty deposits in the arteries seems to be increased by the consumption of saturated fats, but just what determines the level of cholesterol in the blood is still an unanswered question. To complicate matters, besides obtaining cholesterol in certain foods (for example, eggs, liver, shellfish and organ meats), the body also manufactures its own supply of cholesterol. While evidence shows that a diet high in polyunsaturated fats lowers the cholesterol production of the body, a high intake of saturated fats, such as those in meat and dairy products, apparently stimulates the liver to produce more cholesterol.

Research is being conducted to determine the cause of atherosclerosis and measures for prevention. The kinds and amounts of fatty substances other than cholesterol may have more to do with the development of atherosclerosis than cholesterol. It may be that cholesterol is not the real cause, but an individual's hereditary inability to handle cholesterol and other fatty substances is the cause. Heredity may determine why one individual will suffer from this condition and another with similar habits will not.

The food industry has accepted the premise that cholesterol could be a factor in heart problems, and is marketing cholesterol-free breakfast products, unsaturated fats, and polyunsaturated oils. So-called informative advertising has pervaded the media. What is not pointed out in all the advertising is that *cholesterol is necessary to body functioning* (see section in Chapter 3 on Valuable Role of Cholesterol).

Even if we were able to avoid eating all foods containing

cholesterol, our bodies would still produce it from the food we eat. The healthy body strives to keep the level of cholesterol in the blood constant by balancing the amount we obtain from our food plus that which is manufactured in the body, with the amount that is diverted to make steroid hormones, plus that excreted through the intestine along with the bile. This explains why it is so difficult (and in many cases impossible) to lower the cholesterol level in the blood by restricting cholesterol in the diet.

Nevertheless, until further research is more conclusive, the American Heart Association is still urging most adult males to limit their intake of cholesterol and saturated fat. They suggest that the daily level of cholesterol not exceed 300 milligrams. (One egg contains 250 mgs of cholesterol, and a three-ounce cooked piece of beef or pork contains approximately 85 mgs.) So we particularly need to limit our consumption of saturated fats and high cholesterol foods, if blood cholesterol tests indicate there is a need for cholesterol reduction.

In addition to lowering the dietary cholesterol and saturated fat, physical activity seems to be beneficial in keeping blood vessels open and resilient. In consideration of the latter, athletes, then, may be less prone to atherosclerosis.

AN ASPIRIN A DAY?

Aspirin is a truly remarkable drug. Doctors long have known that acetylsalicyclic acid, popularly known as aspirin, will soothe minor pains like headache and toothache, reduce fever, and lessen inflammation of joints. How it provides such relief is still a mystery.

Besides soothing minor aches and pains, reducing fever and relieving inflammation of joints, aspirin has been found also to be an anticoagulant—it hinders the clotting of blood.

In 1956 a research doctor reported that 8,000 patients had taken aspirin in 2-tablets-a-day doses for a period of 10 years without a single heart attack or stroke among them. In support of this finding of the value of aspirin, another researcher, Dr. Lee Wood at the City of Hope Medical Center in California, pointed to the low incidence of heart attacks in patients with rheumatoid arthritis, patients who usually take aspirin on a daily basis. Dr. Wood suggested that men over the age of 20 and women over the age of 40 should take one aspirin tablet a day on a regular, long term basis. This routine, Dr. Wood believes, would lessen the incidence and severity of arterial clotting diseases. Blood sometimes clots while moving through veins, and that is the root of a variety of diseases, including strokes. A stroke occurs when a blood clot blocks an artery that feeds the brain.

Recent research into aspirin's effectiveness in preventing strokes was conducted by the Canadian Cooperative Study Group. A report on its findings was published in the July 13, 1978 issue of the New England Journal of Medicine. Director of the study, Dr. Henry J.M. Barnett of the University of Western Ontario (Canada), concluded that aspirin every day would probably prove to be effective in preventing strokes. This conclusion agrees with Dr. Wood's finding of regular ingestion of aspirin to prevent arterial clotting diseases.

Blood clots consist of microscopic particles in the blood called platelets. When the platelets become very sticky they tend to aggregate into "crowds"—called clots; this is most apt to happen if one eats a diet containing cholesterol rich foods, or if one is under emotional stress, or is a cigarette smoker, or is not exercising regularly.

Aspirin has not replaced the known preventives for blood clots, i.e. proper diet, regular exercise, avoiding tension, and not smoking. All these measures prevent the hardening of the arteries, but the aspirin, which has no effect on this condition of the blood vessels, can prevent the small clots that finally clog the blood vessels. Aspirin reduces the adhesiveness and keeps the platelets from forming clusters and causing blockage.

Dr. George Sheean, noted doctor-runner, enthusiastically

relates that we are moving toward an exciting and unexpected change in our lifestyles, but now—in between the flabby American and the model of perfection that we should some day become—we need acetylsalicyclic acid (aspirin) in small doses to save us. While we are marking time, unwilling (or unable) to make the total commitment to a fitness program, the best advice may be one that doctors used to joke about, "Take two aspirin and call me in the morning."

AMOUNTS OF SATURATED FAT AND LINOLEIC ACID IN SOME FOOD FATS*

Food	Amount	Total Fat (grams)	Saturated Fat (grams)	Linoleic Acid (grams)
ANIMAL FATS				
Pork chop	1 thick	21	8	2
Chicken	½ breast	5	1	1
Beef				
Sirloin	3 oz.	27	13	1
Hamburger (regular)	3 oz.	17	8	trace
Lamb chop	1 thick	33	18	1
Egg	1 whole	6	2	trace
Milk (2%)	1 cup	5	3	trace
Butter	1 Tblp.	12	6	trace
VEGETABLE FATS				
Safflower oil	1 Tblp.	14	1	10
Corn oil	1 Tblp.	14	1	7
Soybean oil	1 Tblp.	14	2	7
Cottonseed oil	1 Tblp.	14	4	7
Peanut oil	1 Tblp.	14	3	4
Margarine (soft)	1 Tblp.	11	2	4
Margarine (regular)	1 Tblp.	12	2	3
Vegetable fats (for cooking)	1 Tblp.	13	3	3

* Compiled from figures in NUTRITIVE VALUE OF FOODS, Home and Garden Bulletin No. 72, United States Department of Agriculture, revised, January, 1971.

16

Energy Sources

FROM CARBOHYDRATES TO GLYCOGEN

If the athlete gets nothing else from this book, I hope he or she will develop a real feeling for the importance of carbohydrates. The foods included in this grouping have been so misunderstood, so ignored, so maligned that an explanation or a reminder of their importance in the nutrition picture is needed.

The sugar in carbohydrate food provides the most efficient and readily available source of energy. It is important for an athlete to realize that the simple sugars from digested carbohydrates are absorbed from the intestinal tract and transported (by the blood) directly to the liver, where the simple sugars are converted to glucose. The body tissues use carbohydrates, in the form of glucose, and what isn't needed is converted to glycogen and stored in muscle tissue and in the liver.

What is important for athletes to remember is that they have only enough glucose and glycogen in their tissues and bloodstream to provide for energy demands for about half a day. Any additional or extra amounts of carbohydrate consumed in the diet are converted into and stored as fat. The body can store an almost unlimited amount of energy as fat, but only limited amounts of glycogen can be stored, ready for immediate use, and that is used up rapidly during fasting or muscular activity. When glycogen is needed, it is converted to glucose and then oxidized to yield energy. Glycogen levels can be doubled and sometimes almost tripled through diet manipulation by first exhausting, then replenishing muscle-glycogen stores. (See "Carbohydrate-Packing" in Chapter 11 of this book.)

If one wishes to facilitate replenishment of glycogen stores, adequate amounts of high-quality carbohydrates should be included in the diet. Enriched breads and other cereal grain products will not only supply the necessary caloric intake but also provide needed vitamins and minerals which are so important in good nutrition.

SUGAR—EMPTY CALORIES

Athletes may be puzzled about the value of sugar in the diet. We've learned that carbohydrates are the quickest and usually cheapest source of energy for sports activities. Since sugar is a carbohydrate, we wonder about all the dissatisfaction with it.

Sugar, in some form, has been present in our diet for a long time. Virtually all the sucrose our early ancestors had came from fruits and vegetables. They dried apples and whatever other fruits could be preserved. Much of their "sweet food" contained other nutrients—while our refined table sugar is a superb example of empty calories. We get only about 3 percent of our calories now from fruits and vegetables and about 18 to 20 percent of all the calories we consume from the empty calories of the sugar we add to our foods. If we get 20 percent of our calorie requirement from sugar, the remaining 80 percent must supply the entire day's nutrients, and this can be a problem for an athlete trying to lose weight.

Sucrose (table sugar) is not a poisonous substance, but besides providing empty calories, it can be addictive. If we have a "sweet tooth," sugar tastes good, and the more we eat rich desserts, the more we want them until weight can become a problem to our health.

Sugar can be a factor in the health of our teeth because it serves as food for the bacteria normally present in the mouth. If food gets packed down in deep grooves between the teeth, bacteria will grow there. One of the by-products of the bacterial activity is a thick, gel-like substance that sticks to the surface of the teeth and hastens the build-up of bacterial plaque. Another problem is sugar sticking to the teeth during the time between brushings. Honey can do more damage to teeth than a sugary liquid such as cola. However, the acid content of soft drinks, especially if one drinks them regularly can affect the tooth enamel and cause erosion particularly at the gum line.

There is no absolute relationship between the amount of sugar consumed and the number of dental cavities one has. Heredity, brushing, acidity of the mouth, diet, and health of teeth are the principal factors that enter into the picture.

We may think of refined white sugar as unnecessary and try to avoid it, but in our eagerness to find a replacement, we wholeheartedly accept brown sugar (the darker the better), sorghum, honey, syrup, or molasses. We learn that these sugars have small amounts of minerals and some vitamins, but they still are empty calories, and they should be used in moderation. As a substitute, enjoy fruits in their natural state whenever possible. It is hard to believe that we eat, on the average, one-third of a pound of sugar daily. When we realize how many foods contain sugar, it is not too surprising.

If you have become a label reader, you may be frustrated in trying to get complete information about sugar from the label of a product. Labels are not required to state total sugar percentage; they only indicate amounts of the various ingredients. Manufacturers can use several different names to avoid putting the word "sugar" first in their list of ingredients. One almost needs to be a chemist to identify the various products listed. Words ending in "ose," such as dextrose or sucrose, indicate sugar; many products also contain "corn syrup" or "corn sugar." By totaling all of the sugar percentages, you can determine how much sugar you actually are getting in the product.

HONEY IS SUGAR

Honey contains two sugars—glucose and fructose. These are the same simple sugars that are present in table sugar. Both honey and table sugar are quickly and easily digested, and their energy in the form of glucose is readily available to the body for use or storage. We perhaps thought of honey as being a little extra nutritious, a health food, so it is a bit disappointing to find out that it is just a sugar with only a very minute amount of available nutrient. It has no special energy-producing value beyond that of other sugar products.

Unfortunately, honey is promoted as a quick-energy supplement for the athlete. Claims for honey products should be analyzed; maybe they are not needed for energy. Money might be better spent for oranges, which have important vitamins, minerals, and carbohydrates in the form of natural fruit sugar.

Remember: honey in excess amounts tends to draw fluid from other parts of the body into the gastrointestinal tract. This shift in fluids, the same as when sugar is ingested, may add to the problem of dehydration in endurance-type sports where sweat loss can be appreciable. No more than 50 grams (3 rounded tablespoons) of honey in a liquid should be taken during any one-hour lapse. Sugar or honey foods do not seem to improve performance in short-term events, including wrestling, except for tournament activity, which may last several hours.

SUGAR BEFORE AN ATHLETIC COMPETITION

Sugar is almost an instant energy source. Refined sugar passes quickly through the intestinal walls into the bloodstream. The product of digested sugar—glucose—is released into the bloodstream faster than it is from other foods.

We should remember that the body has sizable reserves of energy to call upon. Some is stored as glycogen in the muscle tissues, some is stored in the liver, and some is stored as glucose in the body fluid. This is the energy that is used for short-term athletic events. For one who is well-conditioned and has been eating according to good nutrient practices, it is readily available energy. If the athlete eats a small amount of sugar before exercising, the sugar will be metabolized quickly and moved into storage with other energy reserves.

But large amounts of concentrated sugar in the form of honey, glucose, dextrose, or even sucrose should not be consumed immediately prior to an event. These large amounts of sugar can either bring about a hypoglycemic condition or draw fluid into the gastrointestinal tract, contributing to cramps or other problems of dehydration and stomach upset.

The only time the athlete needs to eat some form of sugar to replace the amount that has been depleted is after an hour and a half of continuing steady exercise, such as a marathon run or other lengthy activity. Extra sugar before a single, short-term event gives no particular extra energy—it's already in your body ready to be used.

SNACKS CAN BE IMPORTANT

Many people think that snacks are primarily "junk foods." Some are, but don't be misled. Hamburgers, toasted cheese sandwiches, pizza, tacos, and milk shakes are good food. Money spent for these or snacks of milk, cheese, vegetables, and fruits is well spent *if* the calories are needed. You are the one to decide whether you can afford the calories of a banana split or whether a frosty, low-calorie fruit drink would be a better choice for your daily calorie-nutrients expenditure.

Tests reveal that sugar eaten as part of a meal causes less damage to teeth than the same amount consumed as a between-meals snack. That is probably because the other foods and liquids consumed during a meal help remove the sugar from tooth surfaces.

Snacks can be an important part of your daily quota of calories. They also are important in the social life of the athlete. Enjoy socializing, but plan eating to benefit your health and energy. There are better snacks than potato chips and better beverages than colas.

REFERENCES FOR FURTHER READING

Books

Church, C. F., and H. N. Church. *Food Values of Portions Commonly Used.* Philadelphia: Lippincott, 1970.

Deutsch, R. *The New Nuts Among the Berries.* Palo Alto, California: Bull Publishing Co., 1977.

Guyton, A. C. *Function of the Human Body.* 4th ed. Philadelphia: W. B. Saunders, 1974.

Konishi, Frank. *Exercise Equivalents of Foods; a Practical Guide for the Overweight.* Carbondale, Illinois: Southern Illinois University Press, 1973.

Mathews, D. K. and E. L. Fox. *The Physiological Basis of Physical Education and Athletics.* Philadelphia: W. B. Saunders, 1976.

Williams, Roger J. *The Wonderful World Within You.* New York: Bantam Books, 1977.

Periodicals

Carrol, K. K. "Dietary Protein in Relation to Plasma Cholesterol Levels and Atherosclerosis," *Nutrition Reviews,* 36:1-5 (January 1978).

"Effect of Glucose Ingestion on Substrate Utilization During Prolonged Exercise," *Nutrition Reviews,* 36:37-8+ (February 1978).

Feeley, R. M., P. E. Criner, and B. K. Watt. "Cholesterol Content of Foods," *J. Am. Dietet. A.,* 61:134-149 (August 1972).

Howald, H., B. Segesser, and W. F. Korner. "Ascorbic Acid and Athletic Performance," *Annual of New York Academy of Science,* 258:458-64 (30 September 1975).

Kumnerow, F. A., *et al.* "Influence of Egg Consumption on the Serum Cholesterol Level in Human Subjects," *Am. J. Clin. Nutr.,* 30:664 (May 1977).

Ryan, A. "Round Table—Balancing Heat Stress, Fluids and Electrolytes," *The Phys. and Sports Med.,* 3:43-52 (August 1975).

Sodhi, H., and D. Mason. "New Insights into the Homeostasis of Plasma Cholesterol," *Am. J. Med.,* 63:325 (1977).

Witschi, J. C., M. Singer, M. Wu-Lee and F. L. Stare. "Family Cooperation and Effectiveness in a Cholesterol Lowering Diet," *J. Am. Diet. A.,* 72:384.

part 5

Discomforts

17

Overactive Glands

ACNE

The most common and most devasting affliction, psychologically, among adolescents is acne. Dietary deficiencies, as was pointed out in the chapter on vitamins, are responsible for a number of skin disorders. However, acne is actually the result of a glandular disturbance, although we have long been warned that it is the result of eating chocolate and fried foods.

Cause

Dermatologists recognize that the underlying cause of acne is the reaction of the male and female sex hormones upon hair follicles and oil glands of the skin. As part of the natural growth process, the oil glands of an adolescent increase in size, and although there are wide variations in the amount of oil secreted in different areas of the skin, the most active of these glands are located in the scalp (we are familiar with oily hair), followed in descending order of activity by those in the forehead, face, chest, and upper back. These areas have high oil content, and (except for the scalp) are the most frequent sites of acne.

There are two kinds of glands in the skin—both of interest to athletes. One kind pours out sweat; the other discharges oil. The oil glands, which increase in size at puberty and secrete more oil, are called sebaceous glands. These oil glands generally open into the hair follicles. The follicles, which include a protruding hair shaft, are tiny skin cavities, or tube-like indentations, in the skin. A sebaceous gland secretes sebum (a whitish fatty substance) into the follicle.

The normal follicle is lined with cells that age, die, and are extruded through the pore of the skin. In time, these cells are replaced by younger ones and the cycle continues. In cases of acne, the wall of the hair follicle is thickened and horny, and the older, dead cells accumulate in layers, thus giving rise to plugged pores, which are the direct cause of acne. The "plug" serves as an irritant to the skin in exactly the same way as any other foreign body would. This irritation results in red, inflamed pus pimples or deep cysts.

Acne infection, like chickenpox, destroys skin tissue, and when healed, generally results in permanent scars.

The tendency to acne often runs in families, especially those in which a parent has oily skin. If the overactivity of the sebaceous glands or the plugging of pores could be better controlled, acne might pose less of a problem. The sex hormones, testosterone and progesterone, stimulate the sebaceous glands while the hormone estrogen tends to reduce their activity. Estrogen, however, must be taken in fairly large doses—so large as to produce undesirable side effects in the male—if it is to reduce sebaceous gland secretion to a degree that might be significant in reducing acne.

Whatever the reasons for this gland activity, the oily skin's tendency to acne is aggravated by nervous tension, overwork, lack of sleep, irregular hours, dietary indiscretions, and constipation.

Cleansing Treatment

Since acne is brought about by excessive oiliness of the skin, every effort should be made to keep the skin free from oil. The following points should be observed in this effort:

1. Do not use face cream or grease of any kind.
2. Men may shave but should avoid all shaving products (and shampoos) that contain oil.
3. Wash the face several times a day; there is no actual proof that face-washing helps, but scrubbing with a soapy washcloth does remove some oil and dead skin. Hot water will be more effective than cold water in removing skin oil. Use as "rough" a washcloth as the sensitiveness of your skin will permit. Ordinary soap is adequate for cleansing the skin. (Note comments below on soaps.)
4. Avoid any cream-type cosmetics—the dry kind are preferable.
5. Do not squeeze pimples. One of the prime temptations with acne is to pick and squeeze at blackheads and pimples. Resist it. Handling acne blemishes can spread infections, rupture follicle walls, and lead eventually to deep-pitted scars. (If you feel compelled to remove blackheads, buy a blackhead extractor from a pharmacy. Before you use it, soften the plugged pores by applying warm water compresses for a few minutes.)

Soaps for Acne

There are heavily advertised soaps for acne, but those knowledgeable on this subject consider ordinary soap adequate for cleansing the skin. *Soaps with sulfur* are "good sounding," but it is felt that the sulfur in the soap is not on the skin long enough, nor does it go deep enough to do any particular good. Besides, it is quickly washed away! *Soaps with "antibacterial"* printed on the label sound effective until one realizes that the bacteria live *beneath* the skin's surface, deep within the follicles. They cannot be reached by antibacterial cleansing products. *Abrasive soaps* might have some value for individuals with less tender skin. These soaps contain irritating granules that cause peeling; they can be quite harsh. Experiment by using an abrasive soap once a week and evaluate the results; if pleased, use more frequently. *Tincture of green soap*—long a favorite of doctors and pharmacists—has good cleansing power and is available at your pharmacy.

Medication for Acne

A wide variety of over-the-counter acne-curing products is available. These include creams, cleansers, gels, lotions, soaps, powders, a variety of scrubs, impregnated towelettes, and many other items. There is something for every acne sufferer. Ingredients commonly used in these remedies and believed by most dermatologists to be of some value are:

1. *Retinoic acid* (vitamin A acid)—the most recent addition to acne therapy. Superior to benzoyl peroxide and to a sulfur/resorcinol lotion in producing irritation and peeling. Patience is required; the acne may even appear to worsen during the first six weeks of treatment. Improvement is rarely seen before three to four months.
2. *Benzoyl peroxide*—strong action, creating inflammation and peeling; often results in good improvement.
3. *Sulfur*—preparations should have at least 2 percent sulfur to be effective.
4. *Resorcinol*—remedies with less than 2 percent of resorcinol as their only curing agent are probably too weak to do any good.
5. *Salicylic acid*—remedies with less than 2 percent of the salicylic acid as their only curing agent are probably too weak to do any good.

Avoid products that do not include any of the above five effective ingredients on their labels. Some preparations may list one or more of the five effective ingredients, and the labels do not always specify percentages. If the product does not state the percentage of each ingredient, don't buy it because the percentage of the ingredient may be so low that it cannot be effective.

Because each person's skin differs in sensitivity and each person's acne problem is different, no single acne product is suitable for everyone. If your skin is sensitive and your acne mild, try a formulation that is not as strong as retinoic acid or benzoyl peroxide. Sulfur/resorcinol or sulfur/salicylic acid combinations are possibilities. If your skin is pretty tough and your acne moderate, start with a retinoic acid/benzoyl peroxide formulation. Read labels. Follow directions carefully; keep notes of medication and progress of healing.

If careful trial of over-the-counter medications, thorough skin cleansing, a good diet, plenty of liquids (such as water), exercise, and sufficient rest do not help, a physician should be consulted. One should keep in mind that acne, which may respond slowly even to a physician's treatment, is likely to be even more stubborn with hit-or-miss self-medication.

Antibiotics are sometimes put in over-the-counter creams or ointments; but there is no evidence that such products will prevent, relieve, or cure acne. Read the label and save your money if necessary curing agents are not there.

Ultraviolet rays from sunlight or a sunlamp are helpful in acne when the exposure is sufficient to cause a reddening and slight scaling of the skin, but the danger of over-exposure resulting in severe facial burns often outweighs any benefits. The eyelids are particularly vulnerable to ultraviolet radiation.

X-Ray Treatments

A series of X-ray treatments given by a competent dermatologist will do more to reduce overactivity of the oil glands than anything else. There are several misconceptions about X-rays; one is that they can cause sterility. As used to treat acne, X-rays do not cause sterility.

Dermabrasion

Dermabrasion (plastic planing) of the skin is a way of flattening and improving facial scars by the use of a motor-driven, stainless steel brush. This procedure, which is relatively painless, is performed by a physician or a dermatologist. Usually, the activity of the acne decreases following dermabrasion so that fewer cysts and pimples appear after treatment than before.

Role of Nutrition

In vitamin A deficiency the skin and mucous membranes, including the linings of hair follicles, become thickened and horny. In acne similar changes occur in the hair follicle; therefore, some doctors have reasoned that extra large doses of vitamin A might prevent or cure acne. So far the treatment has been unsuccessful.

Although diet alone will neither clear the skin nor prevent acne, a well-balanced diet is important to skin health. Since nutrient demands are greatest during the growth phase of adolescence, every effort must be made to assure a good supply of calories, proteins, vitamins, and minerals. To deviate from a balanced diet in an attempt to clear up acne is not only foolish but very hazardous.

Most authorities agree that any type of dietary manipulation usually makes no difference in the severity of acne, but with some it seems that specific foods do aggravate the condition. The foods usually implicated in acne are sweets, nuts, chocolate, and fried foods. If it seems that a particular food worsens the acne, try dropping it from your diet and observe the effect (if any). After a few weeks, re-introduce the food and again note the results. If the experiment convinces you that the food is suspect, try to avoid it completely. More likely, you will find that changes in your diet make little difference in the severity of the acne, and that you can continue your regular diet.

Parents can try to help their young people understand the

nature of acne and not dismiss genuine concern as mere vanity. Acne often causes immeasurable mental anguish to those afflicted. The advertisers of many skin preparations for teenagers play on such anxieties in promoting their products. If teenagers have information about acne, they will be far less susceptible to the blandishments of misleading advertising.

Although a case of acne may seem mild and inconspicuous to others, to the young person affected it seems terribly noticeable and embarrassing. It often causes worry, nervousness, shyness, failure to take part in normal school and social activities, and even deeper and more serious emotional disturbances.

DANDRUFF

Advertising campaigns keep the consumer aware of dandruff and the numerous "remedies" to rectify the situation. One would be led to believe that dandruff is a catastrophe.

Most dandruff is nothing more than a normal phenomenon. The skin all over the body sloughs off dead outer cells, and the scalp, even at its healthiest, shows a mild degree of scaling. To this scaling of dead skin are added the normal oil secretions from the numerous sebaceous glands in the scalp— the combination forms dandruff.

Treatment

The best treatment is frequent shampooing. However, there is no basis for suggesting, as some advertisers do, that germs are the primary cause of dandruff and that an antiseptic shampoo is the cure. In general, all over-the-counter dandruff remedies should be viewed with a skeptical eye. If a remedy is really needed, a prescription or recommendation of your pharmacist should be sought.

Remember, most dandruff is normal, and the main purpose in shampooing is to cleanse the hair of sebum (oil), dead skin, scales, and ordinary dirt. Many athletes shampoo their hair once or twice daily; shampooing that often does not harm the hair. In selecting a shampoo consider your particular kind of hair: oily or dry, fine or coarse, damaged or healthy, considerable dandruff or very little. Read the label to better determine what kind of shampoo you need.

Sometimes the production of oily secretions and dead skin scales speeds up until the flaking is definitely excessive. Severe dandruff, which is uncommon, may require treatment by a physician. Its precise cause is unknown, and although it can be controlled, it cannot be completely cured. Brushing does not aleviate dandruff.

Good eating habits, plenty of exercise, rest, and cleanliness of body and hair will all contribute to a healthy head of hair. There is no evidence that *additional* vitamins and minerals added to the diet will control the development of dandruff or affect the quality of hair.

SEBORRHEA

Dandruff often is confused with another scalp condition, seborrhea, in which there is an excessive amount of sebum, causing very oily hair. It is more common during teenage years when the sebaceous glands are extremely active. Sometimes redness and itching are associated with seborrhea; the forehead, nose, cheeks, and even the upper chest are occasionally involved. It is then called seborrheic dermatitis and requires a physician's attention. Shampoos effective against this condition can be obtained on prescription.

18

Common Infections

COMMON COLD

What Is It?

The common cold is not a simple matter; it is characterized by a complex of symptoms, caused by any one of a group of viruses; currently, 80 different cold viruses are known. That is why people can get more than one cold in a year; the immunity to the virus that causes one siege is no help against the different virus (or viruses) that cause the next. The enormous variety of viruses is also the reason why most scientists are pessimistic about the likelihood of ever developing a cold vaccine.

The common cold is one of the most widespread of all diseases. On a typical winter day in January, more than 30 million Americans will have colds at the same time. The total yearly cost of colds in the United States is more than $5 billion. That includes time lost from work, wages lost, and the cost of treating colds and all the other diseases that often follow. (This does not count all the time lost from classwork by students of all ages.)

It is unfortunate that the term "cold" has been given to this common, but uncomfortable, affliction. The name has led many people to infer—incorrectly—that the common cold is somehow caused by a drop in environmental temperature. There is still no evidence that the common cold ever occurs in the absence of an infecting organism. Also, studies have shown that chilling does not predispose one to infection from the cold virus (or viruses).

Scientists believe that the cold virus generally is present in the throat, but it becomes active only when body resistance is lowered. When the cold virus attacks the mucous membranes of the nose and throat, these tissues are weakened and become susceptible to infection by bacteria, which generally are found in the body. The bacteria are secondary invaders, and the virus paves the way for their entry into the mucous membranes. Although they are not responsible for the common cold, the bacteria can initiate a secondary infection that either intensifies the local inflammation present, prolonging the cold, or causes new complications such as sinus infection or ear inflammation.

The common cold is an acute inflammation of the upper respiratory tract, involving the nose, sinuses, and throat. A cold usually begins abruptly, with a sense of soreness and dryness in the nose or back of the throat. Within a few hours the nasal passages feel congested, sneezing develops, and a colorless, watery discharge comes from the nose. Frequently a headache, a sense of lethargy and malaise, a loss of appetite, and vague pains in the back and legs accompany a cold. A fever is rarely present although in children a temperature of 101° F or even higher often develops. Due to loss of the nasal cavity as a resonating chamber, a characteristic change in voice quality also occurs. The eyes, also, may be affected—becoming red and watery—and if the cold affects the throat, there will be redness, hoarseness, and even coughing. The sinuses, which normally empty into the nasal cavity, become blocked by excessive swelling of membranes. The resulting increase in sinus pressure can cause a frontal headache. Swelling in the upper part of the throat can block the Eustachian tubes—the two narrow canals that lead to the ears. This blockage may cause accumulation of fluid and pressure in the middle ear, which can be painful.

The universal complaint of a cold sufferer is "runny nose." Many other characteristics of a cold are common, but most people have their own specific cold "personality." After 48 hours, the cold is usually at its peak. The nasal discharge becomes thick and sticky and some coughing may develop. The cough does not usually bring up much discharge unless the person has a tendency to chronic bronchitis.

At any time during the course of a cold, bacteria (such as staphylococci or pneumococci) can be secondary invaders, bringing on debilitating infections of the sinuses and ears. The old warning that if you don't take care a cold will turn into pneumonia, is hardly ever true; pneumonia and most other infections of the lower respiratory tract begin in the bronchi and the lungs rather than in the upper respiratory tract where the common cold begins.

Colds that persist or recur repeatedly, or which are accompanied by a steady, prolonged fever or chills, may indicate complications, and a physician should be consulted.

Treatment

There is no cure for a common cold except the body's natural defenses. All one can do is make himself as comfortable as possible and try to prevent complications. Treatment of a cold is not very different today from treatment used by past generations. *Get plenty of rest* and keep away from others as much as practical. *Keep yourself warm. Drink plenty of liquids—hot and cold.* Eat a light diet, including good, hot chicken soup, which is one of the best foods you can eat at this time. Aspirin in small, repeated doses generally gives relief from headache, other aches and pains, and fever. In the later stages of a cold, when the discharge has thickened, nose drops help clear the nasal passages. They should not be used more than once in four hours, though, and if the person has a tendency to nasal inflammation, they should be used especially sparingly.

The uncomplicated cold generally lasts from one to two weeks and terminates without special treatment. *The best remedy for a severe cold is rest in bed.*

Medication

Everyone has heard or read of sure-fire formulas for preventing or recovering from a cold. Some people swear by cod liver oil or alcohol or citrus fruit juices or massive doses of vitamin C. This year, just as fifty years ago, Americans (on the average) will suffer two or three colds a year. The cold will last a week or two (a cough or post-nasal drip may linger) regardless of any home remedy, diet, or drug used to head off or treat the symptoms.

Americans spend almost $800 million a year for cold and cough remedies. Advertisers have claimed preventive and curative virtues for vitamins, lemon drinks, alkalizers, antihistamines, timed-release capsules, antibiotics, antiseptic gargles, bioflavonoids, decongestants, nose drops and sprays, aspirin mixtures, laxatives, liniments, inhalers, room air sprays, and a variety of other products. Many of these drugs do neither good nor harm to the cold victim.

Medical advice rarely is required for the common cold, but a cold sufferer needs a prescription of "patience" since most colds last from one to two weeks whether they are treated or not. Some authorities believe that any attempt to suppress the symptoms of a cold may actually prolong the infection.

For physical discomfort and relief of symptoms in the early stages of a common cold, aspirin in tablet form is effective and economical. When the cold has progressed to the stuffy phase, an effective decongestant in the form of nose drops, containing key ingredients listed in the chart below (under

MEDICATION CHART

Function	Key Ingredients
ANALGESIC .... (pain reliever)	Aspirin, salicylamide, acetaminophen, phenacetin, belladonna alkaloids, alcohol.
ANTIPYRETIC .... (fever reliever)	Aspirin, containing medications, are often taken for a cold but are not needed for *all* cold sufferers. When aches and pains accompany a common cold—and a fever also on rare occasions—**aspirin should be taken. However, some cold remedy formulations do not include amounts large enough to act effectively either as an analgesic or an antipyretic.**
ANTIHISTAMINE .... (treat infection)	Chloropheniramine maleate, metapyrilene hydrochloride or fumarata, pyrilamine maleate, phenyltoxamine, thenyldiamine. The inclusion of antihistamines in a cold medication is unnecessary since antihistamines have not been shown to be of value in the treatment of the common cold. **The routine use of antibiotics for colds is definitely discouraged.** These drugs should be taken only in cases with a definite bacterial secondary infection such as broncho-pneumonia, sinusitis, or otis media. Infants and young children seem to be more susceptible to these secondary infections than adults.
DECONGESTANT .... (for stuffy stage)	Phenylephrine hydrochloride, phenylpropanolamine hydrochloride. Decongestant nose drops may provide transient relief for a stuffy nose and might also forestall ear complications by preventing blockage of the Eustachian tubes. Decongestants are more effective when applied as nose drops than when taken orally. Use of nose drops or sprays should be restricted to two or three times a day. They will provide initial relief but actually may worsen nasal congestion (rebound effect) if use is continued beyond three or four days.
COUGH SUPPRESSANT ... (for dry, irritating cough)	Codeine (narcotic), dextromethorphan (non-narcotic), noscapine.
EXPECTORANT .... (for rattly cough)	Ammonium chloride, sodium citrate, ipecac, terpin hydrate, glyceryl guaiacolate, chloroform.
PREVENTION	Vitamin C. There is some evidence to support the claims of the value of vitamin C in preventing or curing (?) the common cold, but more careful testing needs to be done.
MISCELLANEOUS	There are a great many other ingredients, mostly consisting of vitamins and a variety of flavoring agents, that have no known effect on a cold.

"Decongestant") is suggested; but *no medication is necessary if there are no complications to the cold.* The drug industry, nevertheless, has provided us with a maze of products to help(?) us to greater physical comfort.

If you feel the need for an over-the-counter medication, a listing is provided below. On the left is listed the *function* (pain reliever, cough suppressant, etc.). On the right are listed the *key ingredients*—what to look for on the label of the medicine you are purchasing. If at least one of the ingredients is not listed on the label of a decongestant, for example, you will know it cannot do the job you intend it to do.

Prevention

The common cold is an illness that is caused by a virus (or viruses), and it can be transmitted either by direct or indirect human contact or by contact with the materials containing the specific disease-producing agent. Such an illness is called a contagious disease—the common cold is contagious.

The increased incidence of colds in winter probably reflects the fact that much time is spent indoors, thereby facilitating the transfer of viruses from person to person.

The air in our homes can be a factor if it is too dry; the mucous membranes in our nasal passages become dried out, and then the germs can grow and the infection spreads. For this reason, it is especially important to keep indoor air moist in the winter.

Indoor sports events in winter where large groups of people congregate are excellent sources for transmission of infection.

We have thought that the common cold was spread by sneezing and coughing or even kissing, but it is now theorized that the germs of a common cold are spread more by shaking hands and touching or handling contaminated matter. The home, office, classroom, bus, or any other place where people gather is a good spreading ground. Therefore, to minimize transmission of the cold virus, medical consultants suggest that cold sufferers wash their hands frequently and avoid touching their eyes and nose unnecessarily. The use of throw-away paper tissues is a good practice since this cuts down the number of times the cold sufferer handles infected materials.

Resistance to a cold seems to vary greatly among individuals, so not everyone exposed to a common source of infection will become ill. The natural factors, whatever they are, that contribute to resistance in an individual may be operative at one time and not at another.

COUGH

A cough is an act in which air is suddenly forced out of the lungs. A cough is the body's way of removing sputum or any other irritating foreign substance from the throat, windpipe, or lungs. Coughing that is necessary to keep the tubes of the lungs and other air passages clean is helpful. Coughing is accomplished when the muscles of the chest and abdomen are contracted suddenly and send a blast of air out through the mouth. Too much coughing over a period of time can cause great muscle soreness throughout the chest and abdomen and even exact an extra load on the heart.

Coughing is a multiple-stage reflex action that is controlled by a cough center in the brain, which responds to irritation in the respiratory tract. Coughing most frequently is associated with or follows the common cold. Most effects of a cold ordinarily disappear in a week or two, with or without treatment, but a cough accompanying a common cold can linger.

Treatment

Coughing usually can be relieved by sucking plain, hard candies, by drinking hot beverages, or by inhaling steam from a vaporizer. The main purpose of the vaporizer is to put a great deal of moisture into the air and thereby loosen secretions in the upper respiratory tract. This is a safe, drug-free, and inexpensive way to relieve a cough that sometimes accompanies a cold. Any one of these simple measures should limit the frequency and severity of coughing, but any cough following a cold and lingering longer than a week should have the attention of a physician.

Medication

Cough medicines usually have a soothing, psychological effect that relieves the uncomfortableness of coughing. The ingredients in typical over-the-counter cough mixtures that have the most significant effects are *sugar* and *alcohol*. Sugar acts as a demulcent, which seems to relieve sore, irritated mucous membranes, and alcohol acts as a mild depressant of the central nervous system.

Cough mistures, whether over-the-counter or prescription, contain as few as two or as many as ten different drugs, all formulated to act on various links in the cough mechanism. Ingredients are claimed to *decrease* (or *increase*) the secretion of mucus, *stimulate* the sympathetic nervous system, *inhibit* the parasympathetic nervous system, *depress* peripheral nerve reflexes, *depress* the cough center in the brain, *tranquilize* (or *stimulate*) the patient, and *combat* allergies.

Frequently used ingredients in cough mixtures are codeine (a narcotic), controlled by prescription in some states, and dextromethorphan (a non-narcotic similar in action to codeine). These drugs exert a mild depressant action on the cough center in the brain.

The amount of an expectorant in a cough medication is important; otherwise, the mucus secretions will not be loosened and "coughed up." Expectorants in a cough medication include ammonium carbonate, ammonium chloride, ipecac, guaiacolate, potassium iodide, or terpin hydrate, but sometimes they appear in such small amounts that they are not effective in promoting a cough.

Faith in a cough medicine has been found to be important in its use. In other words, when cough remedies work, they usually do so by altering the patient's emotional state in such a way as to reduce the anxiety about the cough and to induce a belief that improvement really has resulted from the medicine. Many people derive great psychological satisfaction from cough remedies even when it has been objectively demonstrated that the remedies failed to reduce either the frequency or the intensity of the cough.

Cough drops and medicated lozenges are popular items in the cough-remedy market. Cough drops contain varying combinations of honey, cocilana, camphor, glycerine, menthol, eucalyptus oil, and flavoring agents. If you feel these medicated drops help your cough, you will be satisfied, but if you would like to experiment, try inexpensive hard candy for something to suck on to relieve a "tickle" or a cough.

SORE THROAT

A sore throat is an inflammation of the throat. In a common cold the soreness is usually in the back wall of the upper throat and affects the nasopharynx and palate. Inflammation is manifested by redness, swelling, and sometimes excessive discharge of mucus.

Once bacteria or viruses initiate an infection, the tissues of the throat react to combat it. Blood vessels dilate to increase blood flow to the area and bring blood cells that act as scavengers. The increased blood flow causes the mucous membranes to redden and the underlying tissues to swell. It is the swelling that is primarily responsible for the soreness. Swelling and inflammation of the throat can produce pain in the ears due to blocking of the Eustachian tubes, which pass from the nose to the ears. A sense of fullness or obstruction, with much spitting and coughing also can develop.

Cause: Bacteria or virus?

The most common cause of a sore throat is infection caused by either a virus or bacteria. It is difficult, but very important, to distinguish between bacteria and viral sore throats in order to obtain the appropriate treatment promptly. Most throat infections are viral rather than bacterial in orgin, but since fever may accompany both types, it will be necessary to consult your physician for diagnosis.

The familiar "strep throat," caused by streptococci bacteria, sometimes can be distinguished by yellowish pus covering the tonsils. Unfortunately for diagnostic purposes, that appearance can be mimicked by certain viruses, such as those causing infectious mononucleosis. Unless there is an allergy history, penicillin is the usual treatment for strep throat. If left untreated, a strep throat (bacterial) can lead to heart or kidney damage. Occasionally, other bacteria such as staphylococci or gonococci can cause sore throats, but streptococci account for most bacterial infections.

If the sore throat should prove to be viral in origin, the consequences are not as serious as when they are bacterial. However, viral sore throats are less easy to identify; culture techniques for detecting viruses are much more complicated. Since a sore throat sometimes is an early symptom of several serious diseases, including measles, scarlet fever, chickenpox, whooping cough, influenza, and diphtheria, it is risky not to check with your doctor.

Treatment

Recommendations for treating a sore throat include the following:

1. *Avoid* over-the-counter remedies.
2. Gargle with warm salt water. Use ½ teaspoon of table salt to an 8-ounce glass of warm water. Use this solution both as a gargle and mouthwash. This mildly concentrated salt solution may help to reduce the painful swelling.
3. Take ordinary aspirin for general discomfort.
4. If the sore throat lasts more than a day or two or is accompanied by fever, check with a doctor.

Caution: Do not crush aspirin to use as a gargle. Gargling with crushed aspirin in water is not only ineffective for the relief of a sore throat but aspirin particles actually can cause injury if they are not swallowed and remain in contact with delicate throat membranes.

Word of Advice: Insistent advertising has pressured many people suffering from a sore throat to accept improbable ideas about the efficiency of gargles, mouthwashes, lozenges, and even medicated chewing gum. Antiseptic gargles and mouthwashes can do little to cure the infection when the invading organisms are deep in the throat tissues—only an appropriate antibiotic can take care of them.

Commercial mouthwashes have no medical advantage over salt water, but mouthwashes can "legally" claim on their label "to help provide soothing, temporary relief from dryness and minor irritations of the mouth and throat." Mouthwashes do not stop bad breath, kill germs, or combat colds.

A Note for Prevention: In winter some sore throats can be traced to insufficient humidity due to overheated houses and closed windows. Dryness of the mucous membranes can predispose one to infections of the upper respiratory tract. A humidifier, an open pan of water, or even several house plants will provide additional humidity.

19
Elimination Afflictions

DIARRHEA

Diarrhea is an intestinal disorder characterized by frequent discharges from the bowels. These discharges are soft at first, and then they become watery. The victim has pains in the abdomen; he is thirsty and sometimes feverish. In severe cases the bowel discharge contains mucous or blood. Diarrhea is a symptom, rather than a disease in itself.

Acute diarrhea can be caused by infected food, infected water, underripe or overripe fruit, highly spiced foods, alcoholic drinks, spoiled meats, or some poisons such as arsenic and mercury; even some cathartics can bring on diarrhea.

Cause

Diarrhea usually subsides after the elimination of the causative material unless the diarrhea is chronic. If chronic, a thorough

218

study by a doctor of the person affected and of the evacuated material is essential to establish the specific cause of the diarrhea. The physician will be interested not only in the patient's physical condition but also in his emotional and mental state, the length of time the diarrhea has existed, the type and location of any pain, and the diet prior to the onset of the condition. The physician will try to establish the specific cause of the diarrhea and direct the treatment toward elimination of the cause rather than just the symptom.

Treatment

If diarrhea is accompanied at any time by fever, severe abdominal pain, or bloody stools, self-medication is not advisable, and the patient should consult a physician. However, a person experiencing diarrhea, but without the preceding complications, may apply the following self-treating procedure:

1. Sip ginger ale, either straight or mixed with a little fruit juice. Sip this slowly from a small glass, taking at least 10 minutes to drink the first small serving. If this causes no upset, wait half an hour or an hour, and then try another small glassful. Continue small servings of ginger ale, fruit juice, weak tea, or clear broth at quarter-hour intervals until the diarrhea has been stopped for at least 6 hours. It is necessary to consume liquids to replace loss of fluids in the watery stools.
2. After at least 12 hours from the beginning of the diarrhea, if you have kept down the above liquids try soft custards, a poached egg, toast, cooked cereal, or bland soups such as chicken noodle or chicken rice (rice is a good bland food to add to the diet).
3. Wait at least 24 hours before you eat ordinary food. If you develop the least sign of nausea, diarrhea, or severe loss of appetite, quit food and liquid again for 4 to 6 hours and start back on liquids.

4. Watery stools wash a great deal of salt out of your system, with the result that you often feel weary and dragged out for days or weeks afterward. Your body has lost sodium chloride and also potassium salts during the diarrhea attack. During and immediately after recovery, plan to salt your food well, and include potassium foods such as bananas and citrus fruits in the diet.
5. If one wishes to try medication, there are some over-the-counter preparations commonly used for acute diarrhea; they contain kaolin/pectin as active ingredients. Read labels to identify whether one or the other is contained in the product. Kaopectate and Pectocil are examples of medications for diarrhea. Follow directions carefully.

Most attacks of diarrhea tend to be self-limited, with the symptoms disappearing (with or without medication) in a few days. The loss of fluids and minerals from the body is potentially very dangerous. If the diarrhea condition persists more than a couple of days, or if there is accompanying fever or vomiting, a physician should be consulted.

CONSTIPATION

Constipation is not a disease—it is a "habit." One of the most common complaints afflicting humanity is constipation, which is the retention of solid waste material within the bowel for an undue length of time.

In the final stages during the process of digestion, the waste material enters the colon as a loose, moist mass, and there the excess water is absorbed by the body. The relatively solid mass of waste material then moves into the rectum where it normally prompts the desire for a bowel movement. Evacuation ordinarily occurs about once every 24 hours, with a wide range of variations among individuals.

Cause

When the urge to defecate is disregarded, the sensation passes. It usually returns again during the day, especially after meals, but if the call is consistently disobeyed day after day, the rectum eventually may fail to signal the need for evacuation. The result can be severe constipation.

Why is the call disregarded? It may be suppressed because one just does not want to be bothered, or it may be the result of a lazy attitude, with resulting poorly developed physical habits; it might be ignored because of the pressure of school or other work; it might be overridden by other and stronger stimuli such as a morning train or school bus to catch; or it might be disregarded because there is only one bathroom for a large number of people. These and countless other reasons often create a situation in which the signal is at first ignored, and later not even felt. When such a pattern has been established, a person may develop chronic constipation, which, as a result, he probably will attempt to remedy by laxatives.

Psychic influences, such as feeling in a hurry or overanxiety, can have an inhibiting effect on regular bowel movements. Bowel dysfunction reflects emotional stresses. The human mind is not meant to grapple with the problems of the past, the present, and the future at one time. You will worry less and accomplish more if you take up problems one at a time. Live in the here and now—not in yesterday or tomorrow. Grapple with the present and the future separately instead of both at once—and forget the past!

Relying on numerous over-the-counter and prescription drugs is another possible cause of constipation. Antacids often are a source of difficulty. Among prescription drugs the most notorious offenders are narcotics such as opium and codeine. Another group capable of causing constipation includes those drugs affecting the parasympathetic nervous system. Among them are antispasmodics, antidepressants, and major tranquilizers.

The misuse of laxatives is another important cause of

chronic constipation. Repeated use of laxatives will in time result in changes in the lining and muscle tone of the bowel. Chronic laxative-users may also unknowingly be depleting their bodies of potassium with resulting muscle weakness.

There are more than 700 over-the-counter laxative products. Surely our widespread misunderstanding of constipation and the drugs used to treat it account for the large number and popularity of this kind of drug.

Everyone does not operate on a once-a-day schedule. It is common to find people in perfect health who regularly defecate twice daily and others who evacuate only once in two or three days. Still other individuals have regular bowel movements at still longer intervals without any impairment of health.

Constipation, then, cannot be defined in terms of missing daily bowel movements, but must be related to each person's normal functioning. Missing a few bowel movements should cause no panic. After a few days, things generally return to normal, and the rhythm is reestablished.

Treatment

Most cases of constipation can be cured without the use of drugs; a change in diet, and a desire to change personal habits can make a big difference. If you suffer from constipation, some rational approaches to treatment are suggested:

1. Stop taking laxatives. Many people are surprised that after a short time the bowels begin to move effectively, without laxative assistance. For temporary constipation, the best thing to do is *nothing*. Let nature take its course, it has a marvelous way of righting the human body.
2. Drink one or two glasses of water half an hour before breakfast or on rising.
3. Drink a cup of hot water with a tablespoon of lemon juice before, or with breakfast.

4. Exercise with some brisk physical activity each day. Walking or jogging each morning confers a sense of well-being and relaxation. The abdominal muscles contracting in the course of running or everyday activities serves to massage the bowel. The regularity of exercise also aids in regular bowel patterns.

5. Eat a varied diet, that contains vitamins, minerals, and a sufficient indigestible bulk to aid in digestion and elimination. Fruits and vegetables provide good, moist bulk.

6. Take in sufficient fluid to prevent dehydration of the material in the colon and consequent difficulty in passing a dry mass. Without adequate residue and moisture, the bowel does not function properly. Moisture is important in the diet of constipation victims.

7. Take time—at the *same time* each day—to encourage bowel movement. After breakfast, or whenever you find the "urge" most frequent, set aside 10 or 15 minutes for elimination. At first, you might rarely have movements at this time, but if you persist, your body will train itself to take advantage of the opportunity. Read, listen to a portable radio, or relax mentally during toileting. Worry and tension clamp your bowel into a stiff, inactive tube. Keep relaxed. Flexed hips help your stomach muscles work better at the toilet; a little 6 inch stool under your feet often makes elimination much easier until the habit has been established. A first step in overcoming constipation is to develop new habit patterns, such as getting up, bathing, having breakfast, and even having the "right" magazine available. The development of an effective habit pattern is often the most successful treatment for chronic constipation.

Need for Fiber (Cellulose)

Fiber, also known as cellulose, comprises the plant's supporting structure. It includes the leaves, stems, roots, seeds, fruit coverings, and also the cell walls.

Fiber is provided in our diet primarily from cereals, fruits, and vegetables, Cereals contain needed bran from the protective layer of the seed kernel; fruits such as grapefruit and oranges have edible membranes; and vegetable fibers come from the stems and stalks of plants.

Cellulose is softened by cooking processes, but the body is not able to digest cellulose as lower animals can. However, cellulose serves a valuable purpose because it provides important bulk against which the contracting muscles of our intestine can push. If it were not for this bulk, the passage of food through the alimentary canal would be poorly controlled. If food is of too liquid a consistency, it moves too fast to be

FIBER IN SOME COMMON FOODS*

	Percent Fiber		Percent Fiber
Sesame seeds	6.3	Bread, whole wheat	1.9
Raspberries, black	5.1	Squash, winter, baked	1.8
Coconut meat	4.0	Beans, lima, cooked	1.7
Bran flakes, 40%	3.6	Fig bars	1.7
Oat cereal, with toasted		Avocadoes	1.6
wheat germ and soy grits	3.5	Strawberries, fresh	1.4
Filberts	3.0	Olives, green	1.3
Raspberries, red	3.0	Cereal, dry: corn, rice	
Peanuts (with skins)	2.7	and wheat flakes	1.2
Boysenberries	2.7	Apple, unpeeled	1.0
Artichokes, cooked	2.4	Carrots, raw or cooked	1.0
Shredded wheat	2.3	Beans, green, cooked	1.0
Dates	2.3	Potatoes, french fried	1.0
Prunes, dried, uncooked	2.2	Raisins	0.9
Popcorn, plain	2.2	Cabbage, raw	0.7
Rye wafers, whole grain	2.2	Grapes	0.6
Coconut macaroons	2.1	Banana	0.5
Puffed wheat	2.0	Oatmeal, cooked	0.2
Peas, green, fresh	2.0	Bread, white	0.2
Parsnips, cooked	2.0	Cream of wheat, cooked	Trace

* Compiled from figures in Watt, B. K., and Merrill, A. L.: Composition of Foods—raw, processed and prepared, U.S. Department of Agriculture Handbook No. 8, Washington, D.C., revised, October, 1975, U.S. Department of Agriculture.

well absorbed. Thus, bulk aids in regularity of bowel movement.

In recent years we have *decreased* our consumption of cereal grains, fruits, and vegetables—especially potatoes—and have *increased* our consumption of animal products which contain less fiber.

Increasing the amounts of fruits, vegetables, good bread, and cereals will help provide the fiber we need to aid digestion and elimination.

FLATULENCE

Flatulence is an excess of air or gas in the stomach, intestine, or both. It is uncomfortable, sometimes painful. Flatulence can be caused occasionally by fermentation in the stomach or more often by eating certain types of foods such as beans, peas, or even cabbage and cauliflower. Most of the gas-forming foods are carbohydrates belonging to the "legume" family.

If being unable to digest beans is a problem, start by eating small amounts until the body becomes adjusted to this food. It is important to cook beans properly for a long time at low heat. That will diminish their flatulence-causing properties.

Although too much gas can create problems of bloating and discomfort, a small amount is helpful in fecal elimination. Both cellulose and gas, as well as the organic acids formed by some carbohydrates, stimulate peristaltic activity.

20

Sleep

Sleep, in addition to nutrition, is one of the most important features in the training regime. Sleep is defined as a state (or period) of complete or partial unconsciousness, normal and periodic, in man and the higher animals.

Most people require sleep just as they do food—on a routine basis, but for athletes in training, particularly runners who have practiced the discipline of "fasting," regular sleep is of *more* importance than food.

If a human goes without sleep for more than 24 hours, he cannot function normally; his ability to remember is affected, and even mild-mannered individuals become very irritable if they have lost much sleep. If a person goes without sleep for 3 days or more, he may start "seeing things" and show other abnormal mental symptoms. Food is important to the body, but a conditioned athlete can do without food for 24 or 48 hours (or even longer), and he will not suffer loss of mental capacity as one does from loss of sleep.

Sleep is the great restorer. Many trainers and team physicians advocate nine hours or more of sleep, even at the college level. No one knows why we need sleep or what sleep does, but we do know that it is part of a natural biological rhythm whereby our body processes slow down and our tensions are at least partially resolved. The question for each individual to determine is how much sleep he or she needs.

During sleep the rate of metabolism (BMR) is at its lowest point, only great enough to keep the vital parts of the body in operation. During this time, blood pressure drops, the pulse rate slows down, breathing is irregular and slackened. Also, the body is less sensitive to pain, light, and sound; even body temperature is somewhat lower than during waking hours.

After seven hours of sleep, the heart rate is in a "resting state," circulation is sluggish, the muscles become flaccid, and the whole body begins to lose its tone. Eight hours or nine or more of bed rest does not give the body more vitality. The longer an individual remains in bed beyond a maximum of nine hours, the weaker he usually becomes.

Research indicates that there is no "normal" period of sleep for any individual. The person himself must discover how much sleep he needs for personal efficiency. Each of us has a particular sleep pattern. To determine yours, go to bed and sleep until you awaken naturally and feel ready to get up. That usually will be after six to nine hours.

The effects of different periods of sleep upon our mental abilities have been tested, and some individuals find that sleeping one or two hours less than the usual nightly allotment improves their mental abilities. By adopting a plan of frequent short rest periods or by napping for one hour (say, between 5 and 6 P.M.), one can add one hour a day to his or her waking life. An hour's nap before the evening meal plus six hours of sleep at night, for a total of seven hours, will be more effective rest for most people than will eight hours of unbroken sleep.

Try a schedule of frequent rest periods—as the heart does. In fact, when the heart is beating at a moderate rate of 70 pulses per minute, it actually is working only 9 hours out of the 24-hour period. Thus, its rest periods total a full 15 hours per day.

These ideas of shortening or adjusting the sleep pattern should be tried by each individual in planning a personal sleep schedule. One should experiment, keeping a record of sleep time and making personal observations of mental and physical reactions to differing sleep patterns. It is important for one to gauge his or her own sleep pattern.

There are two major sleeping patterns observed among people. Some persons have a high body temperature and high efficiency rate in the morning. Others have their highest temperature and efficiency in the late afternoon or evening. Individuals who have a high morning temperature generally prefer to go to bed early at night and get up early in the morning. Those having a high evening temperature generally prefer to work late and then sleep late in the morning. They usually wake up tired if they arise early.

Individuals who have well-defined goals will manage with less sleep than those who are "just going along." Those people who are less goal oriented will spend more time in bed and have greater difficulty in getting to sleep immediately. Also, they may experience sleeplessness (insomnia) because of spending more time in bed than the body needs.

REFERENCES FOR FURTHER READING

Books

Darden, Ellington: *Nutrition and Athletic Performance.* Pasadena, California: Athletic Press, 1976.

F.D.A. Consumer: The Common Cold: Relief but No Cure.

HEW Publication No. (FDA) 77-3029; reprinted from September 1976.

Food and Fitness: A Report by Blue Cross—Blue Print for Health. 2nd printing. Chicago: Blue Cross Association, 1973.

Smith, N.J. *Food for Sport.* Palo Alto, California: Bull Publishing Co., 1976.

Periodicals

Beyer, P. L., and M. A. Flynn. "Effects of High and Low Fiber Diets on Human Feces," *J. Am. Dietet. A.,* 72:271 (March 1978).

"Clinical Nutrition: Vitamin C Toxicity," *Nutr. Rev.,* 34:236-237 (1977).

Family Health Magazine. For subscriptions, address Portland Place, Boulder, Colorado 80302.

Graham, D. M. "Caffeine—Its Identity, Dietary Sources, Intake and Biological Effects," 36:97-102 (April 1978).

"Is Vitamin C Really Good for Colds? *Consumer Reports* (February 1976).

Lincoln, A. "Nutrition Power for a More Powerful You." 7 N. W. Edgewood Drive, Corvallis, Oregon 97330: House of Lincoln, 1975.

"Your Cold and What to Do About It." 2807 Central Street, Evanston, Illinois 60201: American College Health Association, 1971.

part 6

The Female Athlete

21

Nutrients to Remember

Nutrition for female athletes differs little from that for male athletes, but there are a few exceptions: fewer total calories are required, depending upon age, size of the athlete, and activity engaged in; the female athlete's desire for reduced body weight often is exemplified by resorting to extremes of dieting; there is a greater tendency toward elimination of meals and eating "odd concoctions" at all hours; there is greater need for additional iron because of menstruation and because of the female's lower genetic level of hemoglobin and consequent need to satisfy the increased oxygen demands.

The total caloric requirement of boys and girls varies little until puberty because body weight and structure are fairly similar. At puberty some differences develop; then, in early adulthood caloric requirements actually become identical again. The need for the B vitamins—thiamine, riboflavin, and niacin—and almost all other vitamins and minerals is not greatly different for the sexes, except for iron.

Food needs are greatest during a girl's fastest growing years—usually from age 12 through 15. Just as important as the *amount* of food she eats is the *kind* of food. A good, but simple, rule to follow is 3 or 4 servings a day from each of the basic food groups: milk, meat (or alternates), cereals and breads, and vegetables and fruits.

VITAMINS TO REMEMBER

Vitamin A often is referred to as the anti-infection vitamin, and it can be of particular importance in helping to ward off common infections. Vitamin A is also important in development of clear, smooth skin, especially desired by female athletes. No additional amounts of vitamin A beyond the normal requirements are needed. Because teenage girls often cut down on their consumption of bread (and thus butter and/or maragine fortified with vitamin A) and deep green leafy vegetables, the low consumption of vitamin A by teenage girls is a matter of concern to nutritionists.

Vitamin D is a particularly important vitamin for female athletes to include in their diets since it helps the body use calcium and phosphorous to build strong bones. Vitamin D is added to milk. Male athletes easily drink their recommended amounts of milk, but females often omit milk—considering it fattening. Female athletes should drink skim milk that is vitamin-D fortified.

Vitamin C is necessary in the intestinal tract for the absorption of iron. Any girl who eats an orange or half a grapefruit or a variety of fruits and vegetables each day should have no trouble getting enough vitamin C in her diet.

Pyridoxine, or Vitamin B-6, is needed by female athletes because it is important in the formation of hemoglobin. It plays a role in the oxygen transportation scheme in the body and is vital in protein metabolism, the oxidation of amino acids for energy, the breakdown of glycogen to glucose, and the proper functioning of the nervous system.

With this long list of functions, a female athlete needs

awareness of foods that are rich in vitamin B-6 for inclusion in her diet. These include meats (especially liver) and some vegetables, including potatoes, wheat bran, wheat germ, and whole-grain cereals. Athletes should realize that in the milling of flour more than 75 percent of vitamin B-6 is lost because it is contained in the outer covering and in the germ; and it is not added in the enrichment process as are thiamin, riboflavin, and niacin.

Vitamin Supplements should not be necessary in a well-balanced diet of the female athlete. All the vitamins are important because they work together. A lack of any one can interfere seriously with the body's growth and functioning. Adding large amounts of one vitamin can upset the utilization of others. For that reason, it is very important for an athlete to eat a balanced diet, relying on getting all the needed vitamins from her food rather than from supplements.

A MINERAL TO REMEMBER: IRON

A diet adequate in most other nutrients will provide only 6 mg of iron per 1,000 calories. That is only one of several considerations for the adult woman to keep in mind in obtaining the daily recommended 18 mg of iron, especially if caloric intake is below 3,000 calories.

Because of wide differences in the degree to which iron from various sources is absorbed, even knowledge of the iron content of foods does not always give a true picture of its availability. Absorption depends on many factors, including the composition of the diet and the individual herself. It has been determined that an individual who is iron-deficient will absorb 20 percent or more of the iron ingested into the body while a person with normal iron storage averages 2 to 10 percent absorption of iron ingested.

All forms of iron, even metallic, can be assimilated in the body, but if the acid secretion of the stomach is greatly diminished in quantity, it will not dissolve the iron ingested.

When a food is eaten alone, iron absorption is different from when it is eaten as part of a meal. Some foods enhance absorption; the vitamin C of orange juice is an aid to the absorption of iron. Meat and citrus fruit in a meal enhance absorption while eggs tend to prevent the release and absorption of iron. Vegetables and some fruits are fairly good sources of iron, but because the cellulose they contain often interferes, the absorption of iron is adversely affected. Thus, it might be wise to take iron supplements or iron-rich foods separately from bulky vegetables or fruits. Fruits and their juice are rated as generally poorer iron sources than vegetables, but the pulp of fruits such as oranges and tomatoes contains twice as much iron as the juice. Vegetables provide about three times as much iron in the diet as fruits. However, the iron content of vegetables is influenced by soil, so there is a wide range of values reported for the same vegetables.

Raisins and other dried fruits often are recommended for their iron content, but the dried product will have no more iron than the original fruit from which it was derived. If too many calories is a problem, before consuming quantities of raisins (with the accompanying calories), try liver and other meats, green leafy vegetables, molasses, and even pork and beans as a dietary source of iron.

One of the substances that makes iron insoluble and consequently poorly absorbed is phytic acid. This is an organic acid that binds iron and makes it less available to the body. Phytic acid is found in all plant seed proteins and in many roots and tubers. It is neither destroyed by normal processing of plant seed proteins nor altered to any appreciable extent during passage through the human gastrointestinal tract. The effects of phytate are of little concern in a diet in which the intake of animal protein, with its concentrated source of minerals, is sufficient. But in a vegetarian diet in which the concentration of minerals may be less and the phytate content greater (because of increase in cereal grain consumption), the absorption of iron could be a particular problem.

Phytic acid is found in whole-grain cereals, wheat germ,

bran, and legumes such as dried peas and beans. Fortunately, methods of food preparation can help make iron more available. Phytic acid is broken down by yeast; thus, whole wheat and other cereal breads that rise for several hours have more iron available than cornbread and muffins, which contain soda or baking powder and rise quickly. (In milling, white flour has most of the phytic acid removed, but the flour is also low in iron content *unless it has been fortified.*) The iron of oatmeal cereal becomes more available if it is soaked overnight (this also shortens the cooking time) and eaten with milk. Any phytic acid left after soaking combines with the calcium in the milk and "spares" the iron for absorption in the body. All cereals and legumes are improved in their iron-absorption value by soaking in water.

Since women need to replace the iron lost in menstruation, every female athlete would be wise to take an iron supplement, particularly during the days immediately following her period although iron supplements might be desirable throughout training and competition. Female athletes who are deficient in iron have a limited oxygen-carrying capacity, which affects total performance. Periodic blood tests will apprise one of the body's iron needs.

There are many iron salts, both organic and inorganic, such as ferrous gluconate, ferrous citrate, ferric ammonium citrate, ferrous fumarate, and ferrous sulfate, that have been promoted by pharmaceutical firms. No preparation to date has been shown to be superior to ferrous sulfate, which contains 36 percent iron and should be the best value among iron tablets.

Usually, iron tablets will be absorbed into the body more efficiently if a tablet of small dosage is taken *twice* a day rather than a large dosage *once* a day. Taking an iron tablet with orange juice should enhance absorbency of more iron because of the influence of vitamin C, but taking an iron pill in the same meal with a serving of oatmeal may result in less iron utilization. Also, since the cellulose of fruits and vegetables interferes with absorbency of iron, take the iron tablet at times other than when eating foods with lots of cellulose.

FOODS TO REMEMBER

Bread is one of the best of foods for an athlete. It is an important carbohydrate food for energy and contains valuable vitamins and minerals—especially when made from whole or cracked grains rather than from finely milled and bleached flours. Women who are concerned about weight should include *good bread* in their diet but omit the extra calories contained in butter or margarine and jam. Limiting intake of bread in the diet may result in the body not receiving dietary requirements of important B vitamins—thiamin, riboflavin, niacin, pyridoxine, pantothenic acid—vitamin E, and many minerals, including phosphorus, iron, chromium, and manganese.

Eggs are an incredibly wonderful food for anyone but especially for a female athlete. The high quality egg protein is amazingly complete, since an egg contains all of the "essential" amino acids; in fact, egg white is pure protein—without a trace of fat. The egg yolk is a rich source of iron and phosphorus and also contains a significant amount of magnesium, with trace amounts of several other minerals. An egg is also a source of most vitamins—except for vitamin C.

FOOD VALUE OF EGGS

Amount	Weight (gm)	Food Energy (cal)	Protein (gm)	Total Fat (gm)
1 whole egg	50	80	6	6
1 yolk	17	60	3	5
1 white	33	15	4	trace

Amount	Saturated Fat (gm)	Cholesterol (mg)	Calcium (mg)	Iron (mg)	Vitamin A (I.U.)
1 whole egg	2	750	27	1.1	590
1 yolk	2	750	24	.9	580
1 white	—	—	3	trace	0

* Nutritive Value of Foods, Home and Garden Bulletin No. 72, United States Department of Agriculture, revised, January, 1971.

Although an egg is a source of cholesterol, there is no particular danger of cholesterol build-up in blood vessel walls of females until later in life (menopause). Because eggs are such an important food—both for health and beauty—they should not be omitted from the diet. In fact, it is suggested that female athletes consume several eggs a week. If you are really frightened by cholesterol, have your physician keep a close check on your cholesterol level. Other foods besides egg yolks contain cholesterol also.

Gelatin formerly was thought to be a good food for female athletes because it was light and airy and could serve as an extra source of energy. Also, it was hypothesized that gelatin (a protein obtained from the collagen derived from bones, connective tissue, and skin of animals) might be a good source of protein for muscle tissue development. However, gelatin now appears to be of little use in tissue building. As a protein source, gelatin lacks several "essential" amino acids; even if completely utilized, it could not maintain nitrogen balance.

Gelatin is not effective as a food for "beautiful, glossy hair and strong, long fingernails." A normal well-balanced diet is the best guarantee for these "attributes." But gelatin is an easily digested food and acceptable in the athlete's diet.

Gelatins are receiving extensive clinical use for helping to maintain circulating blood volume following hemorrhage, and they also are useful in the treatment of shock.

Sugar has been considered by many athletes and coaches a "quick energy" source immediately prior to competing. That is only true if "immediately" means longer than 15 minutes. The same is true for honey. Even glucose, which is absorbed into the bloodstream somewhat faster than other sugars, requires approximately 15 minutes after ingestion before it can be distributed in the body and serve as an active energy source for the athlete.

It is generally agreed that energy needs for athletic events of short duration (under 15 minutes) can be handled by the body's normal glycogen stores. In long distance events a water or fruit juice solution with glucose helps replenish the athlete's energy stores during the contest.

22

Particularly for Women

SPECIAL CONCERNS

Water. Drinking water throughout the day is important. Women are not in the habit of drinking water as regularly and as much as men. Therefore, women athletes should pay particular attention to their fluid intake. Fluid intake at regular intervals is the best practice. (See Chapter 1.)

Heat exhaustion is more common in women than in men. This may be due partly to lack of drinking sufficient fluids or because of extra adipose tissue. The female possesses about 12 percent more adipose tissue than does the male; it serves as insulation and prevents excessive heat loss from internal organs. The skin temperature of the female is higher in warm weather and lower in cold weather than that of the male. (See "Overheating," Chapter 15.)

Skin is not an independent organ of the body. If we want to improve our skin health, we need to begin by improving our body health. If one has acne or a few blemishes, assume that the body needs some attention in correcting the problem. The skin defends the body against bacteria and viruses; it also functions as a regulator of body temperature. It is tough, flexible, and, most remarkably, it is self-renewing! Develop the habit of cleansing the skin well with soap and water. Greases and creams encourage plugging of pores. If you have oily skin, don't be influenced by cosmetic advertising that touts greases, skin foods, and lubricating creams.

Sleep of 9 or 10 hours a night during the fast-growing years is ideal for a female athlete. As one nears maturity, at least 8 hours is desirable. Try to get to bed at approximately the same time each night, especially on school nights. Sleeping

Menstruation characteristics peculiar to the monthly cycle vary greatly in different women. Although the average period is exactly 4 weeks, or 28 days, some women complete the cycle in 3 weeks and some take as long as 5. In others, irregularity might be usual. Slight variations in the individual cycle are not significant, but sudden major changes should receive prompt attention. Undernourishment and a form of anemia could be responsible; your doctor will be able to advise you.

Girls begin to fatten at the onset of menstruation. That is a danger period for adding "fat cells" that, once developed, stay with the individual for a lifetime. Girls should be counseled about putting on excess weight at this time, when they are developing sexually, leaving the "tomboy" stage, and not exercising as much as previously.

Normal menstruation involves a loss of a varying amount of iron, which can be replaced through good nutrition with particular attention to iron-rich foods, especially before and during the menstrual period. A minority of female athletes have excessive menstrual flow. They not only need to increase consumption of iron-rich foods but the doctor may advise iron supplements because of extra oxygen-carrying needs of the female athlete. The need for iron remains relatively constant for females until they stop menstruating.

A menstrual history should be compiled. Those using intrauterine contraceptive devices, which can increase menstrual blood loss, are in particular risk of iron deficiency. This should be noted in the history.

Another related problem concerns the nutritional effects of birth control pills. Coaches and athletes should be aware that oral contraceptive drugs can cause nutrient deficiencies. A well-balanced diet is especially important to women athletes taking these drugs. Check labels and food charts especially for foods containing vitamin C, folic acid, and the "essential" amino acid tryptophan.

Female athletes usually are normal in respect to menstruation. As a group, they have few aches and pains in connection with this monthly cycle, which may be due not only to good physical structure but to exercise. Athletes report that their strength usually decreases quite suddenly a few days preceding menstruation and remains at a lower level through the menstrual period. One of the special problems facing a woman athlete who is menstruating is simply engendering enthusiasm when she feels "blah."

Levels of female sex hormones (estrogens and progesterone) profoundly affect the female's psychological state. Since these hormonal levels vary widely throughout the menstrual cycle, consistent and significant mood swings characteristic of particular phases of the cycle are observed.

During midcycle, when the estrogen concentration is high, there is a decreased level of anxiety and hostility and a high level of self-esteem. During the premenstrual period, characterized by relatively low concentration of estrogen and progesterone, women are significantly more anxious, hostile, and depressed. In women who take estrogen and progesterone oral contraceptives, thus maintaining a relatively constant level of these hormones throughout the cycle, psychological fluctuations are not as evident.

By being cognizant of psychological fluctuations and their cause, women's coaches should be better able to understand and assist the athlete in achieving her maximum performance potential during actual competition as well as during practice sessions.

Muscles and Strength. Muscle tissue in a woman's body averages about 23 percent as compared to 40 percent in a man's body. Women have a smaller proportion of muscle but a considerably larger ratio of adipose (fatty) tissue than men.

Don't worry about developing heavy, bulging muscles. You won't. The hormonal differences between men and women play a role. Men daily secrete 30 to 200 micrograms of testosterone, a male sex hormone, compared with 5 to 20 micrograms secreted by women. Testosterone seems to be required for extensive growth of muscle tissue in response to training.

The female, it is postulated, has the same potential for strength development as the male of comparable size. The relationship between exercise, muscle mass, and strength is not known. By virtue of his larger, more rugged anatomy, the male usually has greater muscular strength, an advantage he enjoys from childhood on.

Endurance capacity of women is better than that of men although women are inherently somewhat weaker and slower than men. In long-term endurance women have a natural advantage over men. That advantage relates to the extra fat women carry in storage. The hypothesis of a German sports physician is that women's bodies are better than men's bodies at metabolizing fat as a source of energy after they have run out of the usual fuels—carbohydrates and glycogen. So far, this hypothesis has been neither supported nor disproved.

Heart. The heart is about 5 inches long, 3½ inches wide, and 2½ inches thick. A woman's heart weighs about 9 ounces (about 2 ounces less than a man's heart). Thus, women have only 85 to 90 percent of the heart size of a man.

Men between 20 and 30 years old have, on the average, 15 percent more hemoglobin per 100 milliliters of blood and 6 percent more erythrocytes per cubic millimeter. This combination of factors gives men a greater capacity to carry oxygen. When women start training, their hearts grow bigger. There are about 6 quarts of blood in the entire body. When a person exercises, the heart pumps faster in order to supply as much oxygen as the body needs. When exercising stops, the heartbeat gradually slows down.

The heart beats faster when a person is excited because it is rushing more oxygen to the muscles to prepare for activity. If a person is wounded and loses blood, the heart speeds up in an effort to make the remaining blood do extra duty. During pregnancy a woman's heart takes care not only of her own needs but also the needs of the unborn baby—her heart increases its output to 150 - 175 percent of what usually is normal.

Bones of females tend to be more fragile. The wider pelvis in women to provide for childbearing lowers the female's center of gravity.

Goiter is a condition in which the thyroid gland is overactive and becomes enlarged. This gland is located toward the front of the neck between the Adam's apple and the top of the breastbone.

The thyroid gland is one of the most important of the endocrine glands. Its secretions control the rate of growth and the rate of chemical changes in the bodies of both children and adults. The thyroid gland also has an effect on respiration, pulse rate, and brain functions.

Goiter is most frequently caused by lack of sufficient iodine in the diet. It also can be caused by very rapid growth or great emotional strain.

The incidence of goiter is about six times as high in females as in males, and the most susceptible groups are adolescent girls and pregnant women. Practices of limiting the use of *iodized* salt in an effort to control adolescent acne or even restricting salt intake for various reasons should be questioned because of the risk of stimulating the growth of the thyroid gland.

Goiter can be prevented by including seafood in the diet, using iodized table salt, drinking water that contains iodine, or taking iodine in some other form.

In the United States goiter is most common in an area adjacent to the Great Lakes and in the Rocky Mountains, where the drinking water has been found to be low in iodine.

Eating Patterns. Skipping breakfast is not a good practice. Some girls skip breakfast or avoid nourishing food in the mistaken belief that this will keep them trim. It is far better to eat properly and get plenty of exercise. Food eaten in the morning is more apt to be used as energy than that eaten later in the day. (See "Breakfast and Its Importance," Chapter 10.)

Snacks are not harmful as long as they consist of nourishing food. However, the body needs only so much food; that not used is stored as fat. If one consumes 2,600 calories a day and uses only 2,500, one could easily gain 10 pounds in a year. So be watchful of *what* and *when* you eat. If one doesn't exercise to burn up the extra calories, they stay with one in the form of unwanted fat.

Body Fat. The male and female differ quite markedly in their proportions of fat, muscle, and bone. The male is usually taller, heavier, has a skeletal framework that is larger and heavier than a woman's, and has a correspondingly larger muscle mass. It might seem that a man would carry more fat; but, surprisingly, a woman has a larger percentage of body fat than does a man.

Body fat is deposited in two general areas. One area is inside all of the organs needing fat for proper functioning. These are the heart, lungs, spleen, kidneys, intestines, tissues of the spinal cord, tissues of the brain, and the marrow of the bones. The fat in these organs is called "essential fat" and makes up only about 3 percent of a man's body composition; a woman's body contains about 12 percent essential fat, on the average. This larger percentage of essential fat in a female is predominately found in the breasts and other organ tissues, including bone marrow. It is thought that this larger amount of essential fat for women is needed for childbearing and female hormonal functions.

The other general fat storage site is in a layer directly beneath the skin and in tissues around the various internal organs, where it serves to protect them from vibrations, shock, and trauma. This fat is called "storage fat." The percentage of storage fat to total weight for both sexes is very similar, representing about 12 percent of the total weight of men and 15 percent of the total weight of women, on average.

Weight Reduction. Weight reduction programs often are requested by 12- to 14-year-old girls who wish to participate in gymnastics, figure skating, or other sports where a slim figure is desired.

Overweight is a common problem among teenage girls today. Lack of exercise, between-meal snacks, and rich desserts all add up to ugly bulges and rolls of fat.

It is recommended that female athletes have less than 20 percent body fat, but even less fat than that should be the goal for women in events where excess weight could be a serious disadvantage.

If you need to lose weight, do so gradually. A pound or two a week is about the right goal. Many female athletes resort to possibly dangerous fad diets such as the "liquid protein" diet or "high fat diet"; or they simply go without eating. The best way to lose weight is to develop a food and exercise plan and to stick with it. Of course, keeping weight off is the easiest and best way to stay slim.

Dieting Plans. Obesity usually stems from emotional and personality problems, which are associated with eating patterns that have been acquired over a lifetime. These patterns are not easily changed. An obese person usually will try a diet, any diet, no matter how implausible it seems. Usually, the person will lose a few pounds and then return to old eating habits. The problem with most dieters is the person's inability to adhere to a prescribed program. It is also unfortunate, but true, that the shrunken fat cells in the obese dieter remain ready to be filled out over and over again!

Of those persons who successfully lose weight on a particular diet program, more than 90 percent regain the weight they once lost. Most of them are ready to try the next diet scheme that comes along: the grapefruit diet, the drinking man's diet, the air force diet, the Atkins diet, the water diet, the Mayo diet, the lazyman's diet, the sex diet, the ice cream diet, the low-calorie diet, the rice diet—the list could continue, but more than mere mention will be made of the latest diet scheme, the liquid protein diet. This diet has attracted much attention among dieters, and others, and has prompted much investigation and charges of poor nutritional practices. Illness, and even deaths, have been attributed to its use.

Liquid Protein is one of the latest weight-reduction products to be marketed. It is sold without a prescription, and there is a real potential danger if the liquid pre-digested protein diet is taken without medical supervision. Dieters are instructed to consume only a few ounces of the liquid protein daily and nothing else. Liquid protein drinks contain about 60 calories in a 1-ounce serving. On the liquid protein diet, women consume 3 to 5 ounces a day and men, 4 to 7 ounces. Since none of the liquid protein diets (there is a choice) is nutritionally complete, use of the diet without any supplementary food can, and often does, lead to serious nutritional deficiencies.

Liquid proteins are made from specially treated (usually referred to as "hydrolized" or "pre-digested") collagen or gelatin, which are obtained from animal hides, tendons, and bones. These products are intended as protein supplements. Some of the liquid proteins on the market are fortified with a limited number of "essential" amino acids, vitamins, and minerals; but *none is nutritionally complete.*

The theory of the reducing benefit of liquid protein as the principal item in the diet is that the consumption of this form of protein alone—without benefit of any carbohydrate eaten in other foods—will maximize the burning of body fat while conserving muscle tissues, which are predominantly protein.

The Federal Drug Administration is inspecting plants and testing liquid protein products to find *how* the products are made and *what* they consist of. Then label claims are checked for accuracy.

People are warned not to use the liquid protein diet without medical supervision. Also, while on the diet, one must remain alert for any warning signs of cardiovascular disorders. Since none of the liquid protein diets is nutritionally complete, medical supervision is important. Vitamin and mineral supplements may be required. A particularly crucial mineral is potassium, not too much and not too little, because a potassium imbalance can cause fatal heart irregularities.

Dieters resuming the intake of solid food after a liquid diet must make gradual adjustment to more normal eating; the potassium and fluid balance especially must be considered, and medical supervision is important at this stage also.

People with kidney, liver, or heart disease or high blood pressure, as well as pregnant women and nursing mothers, are urged not to use the liquid protein diet.

Research is in progress at several medical centers to determine if there is merit in the theory that a person consuming 500 calories on the liquid protein diet will lose less lean body mass (muscle) than a person on another type of 500-calorie diet. This research is concentrated on extremely obese people who are using the diet under strict medical supervision as part of a total program of weight reduction. It is not a program for a do-it-yourself dieter who wants to lose a few pounds quickly in order to "make weight" to qualify for a sport.

The Federal Drug Administration suggests that anyone who wants to lose less than 20-25 pounds should avoid diets such as the liquid protein diet, which involves a "modified-fasting" regimen.

Gaining Weight takes planning to supply more calories than one needs. Usually, the person who is truly trying to gain weight has to work as hard as the one who is attempting to lose weight.

When a female athlete speaks of wanting to gain weight, we assume she wants to gain muscle and not fat. A pound of muscle contains 600 calories and a lot of water, but just eating 600 calories will not build muscle. One must exercise the particular areas where one plans to build muscle; a program of exercise is needed to stimulate the growth. Although most women, because of hormone differences, cannot develop large muscles as men do, they can develop and strengthen muscles with the proper exercise program.

In order for a girl to calculate her energy need, she will need some additional figures besides her present weight. A scale of the suggested number of calories per pound of body weight per day has been worked out according to age groups. These are:

	Age			
	10 years	11-14 years	15-18 years	19 years
Suggested calories per pound per day	33 calories	31 calories	26 calories	20 calories

To calculate energy needs, multiply present weight by the calories per pound needed. Then add some calories to gain on: 500 extra calories a day would result in an average gain of a pound a week.

For example, Mary is 15 years old, weighs 112 pounds, and wants to gain; so she calculates her energy need:

26 calories per lb. × 112 lbs. = 2,912 calories (rounded to 2,900 calories)

Then she adds 500 calories a day to gain on:

2,900 + 500 = 3,400 calories

That is Mary's daily calorie allowance and should permit her to gain 1 pound a week. With this calorie amount, she can plan her daily diet to get the fats, carbohydrates, proteins, vitamins, and minerals that she needs for growth and health.

Good Posture, physical fitness, and attention to a well-balanced diet all work together for a top-notch figure.

Common causes of poor posture are excess weight and flabby muscles, particularly in the abdominal region. Exercise and proper food can help reduce weight, and appropriate exercise can also help strengthen flabby muscles. When one stands and sits erectly, the internal organs have plenty of room, the blood circulates freely, and one can feel on "top of the world!"

Mental Attitude. The state of the athlete's mind can make or break her. Women react to intelligently planned training in the same positive ways that men do, and they break down under excessive loads for the same reasons. They need reassurance; they like attention, they can be fiercely independent, and once their goals have been set, they can be dedicated toward that achievement.

Female athletes know there is nothing as specific in life as a measurement in sports. The height of a jump, the time of a run, or the record broken—all are marks of personal achievement for the world to see. The successful athlete confidently says, "I never let my mind think that I won't do it! I keep my mind always on target." *The dedicated female athlete is an exceptional woman.*

CONCLUDING COMMENTS

The female athlete enjoys and appreciates her body and herself, and she admires the proportions of the physique she was given.

She marvels at the coordination of mind and body in locomotion, and she studies the miracle of how food becomes energy and allows her the opportunity of realizing her vast potential.

She is challenged to care for the marvelous human machine that is her body. Wherever she goes, her body mirrors her. Meticulous care says, "I'm concerned about my health, my posture, my mind, my talents.

"Altogether, it's me, and I care about what my body can do."

REFERENCES FOR FURTHER READING

Books

Guthrie, H. A. *Introductory Nutrition.* 3rd ed. St. Louis: C. V. Mosby Co., 1975.

Klafs, Carl E., and M. Joan Lyon. *Female Athlete.* St. Louis: C. V. Mosby Co., 1973.

Lowenberg, Miriam E., and others *Food and Man.* New York: Wiley, 1974.

Mayer, Jean. *Human Nutrition.* Springfield, Illinois: Charles C. Thomas, 1972.

Roe, D. A. "Nutrition and the Contraceptive Pill" in *Nutritional Disorders of American Women.* New York: Wiley, 1977.

Periodicals

"Bazaar's Action Sports Guide: Symposium," *Harper's Bazaar,* 110:84-91+ (May 1977).

Beaton, G. H., M. Thein, H. Milne and M. J. Veen. "Iron Requirements of Menstruating Women," *Am. J. Clin. Nutr.,* 23:275 (1970)

"Bread Diet," *Family Circle* (November 15, 1977).

Darden, Ellington. "Strength Building Program for Female Athletes," *Woman Coach* (March-April 1975), 161.

Eisenberg, Dr. Iris, and Dr. W. C. Allen. "Injuries in Women's Varsity Athletic Programs," *The Phys. and Sports Med.,* 6: 112-20 (March 1978).

"The Function of Vitamin E As an Antioxidant," *Nutrition Reviews,* 36: 84-6 (March 1978).

Kaplan, J. "Are Girls Catching Up to Boys in Sports?" *Seventeen,* 35:112-13+ (December 1976).

Mayer, Jean. "How to Eat to Feel Your Best," *Family Circle* (September 1975).

Weber, M. "Muscles Do More Than Move You Around," *Vogue,* 168:325-6 (April 1978).

part 7

Energy and the Athlete

23
Energy Demands
of the Athlete

We used to think that all athletes perform at top efficiency on a "well-balanced diet." However, a more complete understanding of energy metabolism indicates that different types of sports activities depend on different energy-producing systems, and these are affected by diet.

The chemical reactions that take place in the body are part of an intricate, delicately balanced combination of interacting energy cycles. We don't know just how these energy cycles interact, but we do know that the body does not switch in and out of succeeding energy systems, turning off one source as it moves on to the next. There occurs, rather, a smooth phasing with overlapping of one energy source into another, as the energy demands increase during any given athletic event.

ENERGY SOURCES

Adenosine Triphosphate (ATP)

The immediate source of energy for muscle activity is a compound called *adenosine triphosphate*, or simply ATP. This is a product formed in the muscles by the metabolism of carbohydrates, fats, and to a much lesser degree, proteins. ATP consists of one molecule each of adenine and ribose, called *adenosine*, combined with three phosphate molecules each consisting of phosphorus and oxygen atoms. ATP is the fuel which all muscle cells need in order to do their work. It can be rapidly metabolized to meet the needs of sudden outbursts of activity in intensive, short-term exercise. When the ATP compound splits off one or two phosphate molecules, the chemical-bonding energy is released in the absence of free oxygen. This is an *anaerobic* energy-releasing reaction, and it is this capacity to provide energy anaerobically (i.e. without free oxygen) that enables the cells to generate energy for immediate use. This is important in strenuous exercise, where the heart and lungs cannot deliver oxygen quickly enough to the muscles.

Creatine Phosphate (CP)

Since the body stores only enough energy to allow one to run as fast as possible for only several seconds, ATP must be resynthesized to provide a continuous supply of energy. Creatine phosphate (CP), another energy-rich compound in the body, is similar to ATP in that energy is released when the phosphate molecule bond is broken by chemical reactions controlled by special enzymes. Cells store CP in considerably larger quantities than ATP, and it is a source of energy for resynthesis of ATP. Thus, CP is considered the reservoir of high energy phosphate, but the energy released from the breaking-off of the energy-rich phosphates from ATP and CP is limited and will sustain all-out exercise such as running or swimming sprints for approximately only 5 to 8 seconds. Thus the capacity for conversion of energy from the phosphate pool (ATP plus CP), and the size of the pool may be important factors in determining a person's ability to maintain speed over a very short distance. Since vigorous exercise depletes the small stores of ATP-CP, the body must turn to another source of energy supply in order to recharge the ATP-CP system.

Glycogen

Another energy source is glycogen, a storage carbohydrate which the body makes from glucose (a simple sugar) and stores in a limited amount in the liver and muscles. When ATP-CP energy has been exhausted (through exercise), glycogen can be metabolized within the muscle cells to restore the supply of ATP. Glycogen is a source of energy for heavy exertion lasting a few minutes. A good nutrition program should be combined with proper conditioning and training to ensure maximum glycogen storage. (See Carbohydrate Packing in Chapter 1 and A Balanced Diet, in Chapter 10.)

Carbohydrates: An Anaerobic Energy Source

Carbohydrates are the only food group that can provide energy anaerobically for the formation of ATP. When glucose enters a cell to be used for energy, it undergoes a series of chemical reactions known as *glycolysis*. During the process of glycolysis, two new molecules of ATP are produced due to the transformation of the original six-carbon glucose molecule to two three-carbon molecules of pyruvic acid. This breakdown occurs within the intracellular fluid medium of the cell. The bonds that chemically bind the glucose molecule together are broken, and hydrogen atoms are stripped away from the glucose molecule. The ATP produced during glycolysis provides a rapid, though limited, source of energy for muscular activity, which is often needed by the athlete who is giving "his all" in that final spurt for victory. The cells' capacity to maintain glycolysis is crucial during physical activities that require a sustained, all-out effort for periods of up to 60 seconds. The anaerobic energy from glucose can be thought of as a reserve of *rapid* food energy for the resynthesis of ATP. The anaerobic reactions of glycolysis releases only about 5 percent of the energy contained within the glucose molecule, but an additional means for extracting the remaining energy is available.

Carbohydrates: An Aerobic Energy Source

As the athlete continues to exercise, he progressively depletes the stores of ATP-CP and muscle glycogen, and the body has to resort to another source of energy. The final fuel available comes from the aerobic metabolism of carbohydrates (glucose) and fats, and a very small amount from proteins. It is extracted when the pyruvic acid molecules from the reduction of glucose through glycolysis are converted to a form of acetic acid, called *acetyl Co-A*. This process releases hydrogen atoms and carbon dioxide gas. Acetyl Co-A then passes into what can very simply be called "energy factories" within the cells, where over 90 percent of the total ATP is produced. Within the cell's "energy factories" when carbon and hydrogen atoms are stripped from the molecules of acetyl Co-A, two molecules of ATP are regenerated for energy, 16 additional hydrogen atoms are set free, and four molecules of carbon dioxide gas are formed.

In a succeeding series of chemical reactions, hydrogen atoms are changed into electrically charged particles (ions) and combined with oxygen to form water. This is the most crucial phase of energy metabolism because it is during the transfer of the electrons from hydrogen to oxygen that energy is produced to drive the rebonding of phosphorus so that adenosine diphosphate (ADP) becomes adenosine triphosphate (ATP).

FAST- AND SLOW-TWITCH MUSCLE FIBERS

Two types of muscle cells have been identified; each has a distinguishing and predominant capacity for energy metabolism, and they are designated as *fast-twitch* and *slow-twitch* muscle fibers. The fast-twitch fiber has a high capacity for anaerobic energy release and is activated during quick bursts of activity, while the slow-twitch muscle fibers generate sustained aerobic energy and are activated in continuous, steady-pace exercise.

EXERCISE AND OXYGEN NEEDS

During steady-pace exercise, the oxygen consumption levels off at a point where aerobic metabolism balances the energy demands of the working muscles. If the exercise intensity exceeds a steady pace, and the requirement for oxygen exceeds that available, then the anaerobic reactions of glycolysis must supply the additional energy. Under these conditions, more hydrogen is produced than can combine with oxygen to form water. However, pyruvic acid from the breakdown of glucose takes up the excess hydrogen to become lactic acid, which is carried away in the bloodstream. This allows the reactions of glycolysis to proceed temporarily to resynthesize ATP, but in a short time, as the lactic acid level in the blood and muscles increases, fatigue sets in and exercise must stop. During rest periods, if sufficient oxygen is available, lactic acid converts back to pyruvic acid and can be used as an energy source through the acetyl Co-A route.

Since the ability to maintain a steady pace is so important in long term exercise, physiological conditioning for endurance must be geared toward the improvement of maximum oxygen capacity. Even under conditions of a steady-pace state of exercise, fatigue will occur if the body's carbohydrate reserves, particularly muscle glycogen, reach low levels. Maintaining an adequate daily intake of carbohydrates is important to top physical performance or conditioning.

If exercise is moderate and predominantly aerobic, or if intense exercise is brief and stops before lactic acid accumulates, recovery will be rapid and exercise can begin again after only a brief rest period. With the proper application of such intermittent or interval exercise, a person can accomplish large amounts of intense work that would normally be exhausting in a few minutes if done continuously. The key to successful training is to identify the predominant means of energy metabolism required for a desired activity, and to train specifically to supplement the kind of energy output needed.

DIET MANAGEMENT FOR DIFFERENT LENGTH EVENTS

The Short-Term All-Out Effort

In preparation for the short-term contest, an athlete should eat foods to supply him with adequate nutrition for his body and energy needs, and also to be assured that muscle sources of ATP-CP and glycogen are sufficient for the up-coming sport activity.

The short-term, all-out effort will depend primarily on the anaerobic metabolism of ATP-CP stores in the muscle cells. The principal considerations for these events are a good supply of water, an adequate diet of carbohydrates and proper rest between contests to build up ATP-CP stores.

Experienced athletes have often met these needs by limiting food intake on the day of competition to frequent drinks of fruit juice or plain water. (A small amount of additional sugar or honey can be added to water if the individual desires and can tolerate such concentrations of sugar. Hard candies and water are preferred by some successful athletes.) Complete liquid meals are increasing in popularity with many athletes who can enjoy a light meal that is convenient and palatable. Also, during track and swimming meets, and during tennis and wrestling tournaments, for example, where competitors are often involved in several daily events, time should be allotted between contests for replenishing glycogen and ATP-CP supplies. (See Chapter 12.)

The Intermediate Length Event

Many of our most popular athletic contests demand intense

muscle exertion for periods of from three to five and up to ten minutes—and some even longer. The mile run, the middle-distance swimming event, the wrestling match, and the rowing contest, to name a few, all demand maximum exertion for short periods and are classified as intermediate-length competition.

Because the anaerobic (without oxygen) energy available through ATP-CP is exhausted after a matter of a few seconds, the energy for intermediate length competition comes from the anaerobic metabolism of glycogen stores in the muscles. Normal levels of muscle glycogen are usually adequate to provide the energy to sustain exercise for intermediate length competition. Ample stores of glycogen can be assured by eating approximately 50 percent (or even a little more) of the daily caloric intake as carbohydrates. If the energy demands of daily exercise are high, increase the carbohydrate content of the diet, but remember to get an adequate amount of protein and fat also. By eating a high-carbohydrate diet (see "High Carbohydrate Menus" in Chapter 11) during the week preceding competition, the athlete's glycogen level can be almost tripled. For many this amount of carbohydrate in the diet has proven successful in improving performance in the mid-length contests.

The Endurance Event

All the energy sources mentioned previously will be used to meet the needs of prolonged effort in the endurance event.

The athlete will use the anaerobic (without free oxygen) metabolism of ATP-CP stores in the muscle cells, and needs sufficient liquids during his endurance activity. He will need to increase carbohydrate intake to supplement glycogen stores in the muscles and may be interested in carbohydrate packing during the week prior to the athletic event in order to provide maximum stores of glycogen. The large stores of muscle glycogen and the extra supply of anaerobic energy will be an early advantage for an endurance athlete. Many endurance athletes consume so-called rice and spaghetti diets in order to achieve a high level of carbohydrate intake.

The combination of diet and exercise to produce a glycogen packing should be of considerable interest to the endurance athlete, especially the marathon runner and swimmer whose success depends partly on the magnitude of the body's carbohydrate reserves. The carbohydrate packing is particularly helpful when intensive output is required for more than 10 to 15 minutes without rest.

It should be pointed out that carbohydrate packing is not equally beneficial to all athletes. It should be undertaken only after experimentation early in the training season, so each athlete will be familiar with his or her reactions to it. Some athletes will skip the first phase of the carbohydrate packing and plan for an increase of carbohydrates in their diet for just the two or three days preceding competition. The carbohydrate packing diet requires knowledge and dedication on the part of the participating athlete. The most difficult part for most individuals is the first phase, with its restricted carbohydrate intake during a period of intensive training, which can leave the athlete feeling weak and lackadaisical. The high carbohydrate diet later in the week preceding competition is easier to maintain. For most athletes, it is advisable to limit the carbohydrate packing diet to important competitions. For less crucial contests, a limited plan can be followed, simply utilizing the high carbohydrate intake two to three days preceding the athletic competition. (Note: the wisdom of a prolonged high-carbohydrate diet has yet to be verified.)

During the day of tournament or marathon competition, athletes will find that lightly sweetened fruit juices (not fruit drinks) are particularly helpful for maintenance of fluid intake. Many fruits also are a source of electrolytes. The electrolyte, magnesium, is important as an activator of various enzymes, especially those which bring about the linking of phosphate groups to glucose in the formation and breakdown of glycogen and the release of energy. It is essential for the reaction of "high-energy phosphate groups," as in adenosine triphosphate (ATP).

Care must be taken in choosing high-carbohydrate foods during the day of competition. Carbohydrates taken in too concentrated a form, as in undiluted honey, can cause a gathering of large amounts of water in the upper gastrointestinal tract, with resulting discomfort and diarrhea. A tense, nervous athlete is apt to have a poorly functioning stomach anyway and may be particularly vulnerable to high concentrations of carbohydrates. Diluted sweetened fruit juices, or fruit-flavored noncarbonated drinks are best tolerated with no more than a ten to fifteen percent concentration of carbohydrate.

The salt needs of even a marathon runner competing in warm weather rarely exceed the amount obtained from a normal diet. Too much salt is actually more of a problem than too little. Too much salt can contribute to heat-related problems. Maintaining a liquid balance and avoiding excessive increase in body temperature are of far greater concern than a threat of salt depletion. The water requirements for endurance competition demand constant attention, particularly in warm, humid weather. Plan for an hourly intake of water beforehand and continued intake at appropriate intervals throughout the event. (See "Amount of Water" in Chapter 1 and "During the Competition—Water Is Needed" in Chapter 12).

Since the metabolism of food and the resulting release of energy in the body is an extremely complex subject, the reader may wish to delve deeper in the subject in advanced texts that include this information. The author suggests the following:

Nutrition and Physical Fitness, Bogert, Briggs & Calloway, 9th edition, W. B. Saunders Co., Philadelphia, Pa., 1973.
Nutrition, Weight Control, and Exercise, Katch, Frank I., and McArdle, William D., Houghton Mifflin Co., Boston, Mass., 1977.

24

The Energy Demands of Specific Sports

BASKETBALL

Basketball requires overall strength in every major muscle group; it is strenuous exercise, and of intermediate duration. The game is often very intense, and for the spurts of energy needed, the major source comes from the anaerobic process of glycolysis. As the activity increases and time of game lengthens, there will be increased formation of lactic acid. If the rest periods at that time are adequate, the abundance of lactic acid may be utilized as a form of energy through conversion back to pyruvic acid. Because of the intensity of game play, as well as length of play, it is desirable that the athlete possess a capacity for both anaerobic and aerobic metabolism.

Players should eat a well-balanced diet throughout the season. Follow pre-event eating schedule at the beginning of Chapter 12. Pay particular attention to liquid intake. The liquid pre-game meal (Chapter 12) is excellent for pre-game nourishment.

BASEBALL

A baseball player needs overall strength in every major muscle group. In baseball the athletic performance is usually of short duration and high intensity when a player catches a ball, hits a ball, runs bases, etc. Energy for this kind of activity comes exclusively from anaerobic (without free oxygen) sources, which are the high energy phosphate compounds, ATP and CP, stored within the specific muscles that are activated in the game. Some baseball plays represent intense exercise for several seconds, which is a blend of metabolic energy demands where a capacity for both anaerobic and aerobic (with free oxygen) metabolism is experienced. The athlete should eat a well-balanced diet throughout the season. Pre-event eating suggestions begin in Chapter 12.

BICYCLING

Bicycling is one sport where men and women are considered to be well matched since leg strength relative to body weight is roughly equal between the sexes.

Cycling performances of long duration require a fairly constant aerobic energy supply. However, bicycle road-racers must have both anaerobically and aerobically derived energy in their long races. For sudden spurts of speed-riding or climbing, anaerobic derived energy is necessary. Cycling about thirteen miles per hour will use as high as ten calories per minute.

Bicyclists should eat a well-balanced diet throughout the season. Eat sufficient carbohydrate foods to provide for essential energy needs. Provide for liquid needs throughout cycling times. The long distance bicyclists often carry their own drinks as they ride and thus have access to a drink whenever they want. (See "Exercise Drinks" in Chapter 14.)

CREW

Regular Crew

Crew members are usually in training throughout the school

year—September through June, with competition generally during the spring months.

Follow a good basic diet throughout the training period. There should be some fluid and carbohydrate intake within a couple of hours before heavy workouts.

Rowing in competition is a most intense energy-expending sport. Carbohydrate packing (Chapter 11) can be helpful to athletes out for crew. Since crew racing is a performance of long duration it requires a fairly constant aerobic energy supply. Anaerobic energy will be needed also for times of extra effort experienced at the finish line.

Light-Weight Crew

Light-weight crew is a weight-control sport. See information on weight reduction and control beginning in Chapter 9. Nutritionally sound solutions to weight problems are necessary for excellent health and effective competition.

FOOTBALL

Football is a sport that requires greater-than-average strength in all major muscle groups. Certain positions in football require tremendous body mass and most players have extra fat to help in protecting vital organs.

Football players need to be particularly conscious of their water intake, and be extra concerned about this in warm, humid weather. See suggestions on pre-event eating in Chapter 12 for both food and liquid suggestions.

Football is basically a performance of short duration and high intensity where ball carrying, kicking, etc. are activities of a limited time. Energy for this kind of activity comes from anaerobic sources, ATP-CP, stored within the specific muscles that are used. The activity is a stop-and-go, on-and-off variety. Some football plays represent intense exercise for several seconds, which then becomes a blend of metabolic energy demands where a capacity for both anaerobic and aerobic metabolism is experienced.

Football players need to be concerned about weight control after their football playing days have ended. Lack of a trim body in later life is a particular health problem for the former football athlete who has not had to limit his daily calories.

GOLF

Golf is considered more of a power game now since the fairways are longer than they were in the early days of golf. Also, the shafts of the clubs are metal in place of wood, and the golf swing formerly was mainly with the arm, but now, in order to get the maximum drive, the individual must use his entire body. Formerly, the golfer needed to concentrate on development of the upper body; now the enlightened athlete-golfer develops the entire body.

Basically, the energy requirement in golf is of short duration and high intensity because the golf swing requires an immediate supply of energy. This energy is provided exclusively from anaerobic sources, specifically the high energy phosphate compounds, ATP-CP, stored within the specific muscles activated in the process of walking or stroking.

Golf strokes require about five calories per minute, and walking requires from three to five calories per minute—depending on how briskly one walks.

GYMNASTICS

Although both men and women participate in this sport, it is felt that girls seem to have a little more skill in standing on one foot or walking on a narrow beam. However, diet-related problems are far more common among women who would like to be successful gymnasts. It is recommended that female athletes should have less than 20 percent body fat, but even lower amounts should be attained in those events where excess weight could prove to be a disadvantage. Excess body weight is not functional; in fact, fatness is considered a real handicap for a gymnast. A weight reduction program, see Chapter 9, can be helpful for one wanting to lose some extra pounds. The upper body development is a particular need for the gymnast.

For strenuous exercise lasting several minutes, which gymnastic routines usually do, the major source of energy comes from the anaerobic process of glycolysis. Intense exercise of an intermediate duration represents a blend of metabolic energy demands. Thus it is desirable to possess a high capacity for both aerobic and anaerobic metabolism.

HIKING

Hiking is enjoyed by more and more women—as well as men. Scheduled food and liquid replenishments are essential for optimum energy and actual enjoyment. Concentrated sources of carbohydrates (see the beginning of Chapter 16) are ideal for energy, especially if the hike is a prolonged one. Performance of long duration requires a fairly constant aerobic energy supply.

JOGGING

Jogging has become a popular form of exercise. It is felt that running-jogging is a relatively safe activity for all ages and both sexes, but especially good for the middle-aged adult! About the age of 35 years, many people realize they are beginning to slip—gain weight, lose agility, lack endurance, and experience a cardiac-respiratory decline. Only a few weeks of jogging brings a noticeable improvement in physical as well as mental well-being.

Performances of long duration, such as recreational jogging, require a fairly constant aerobic energy supply.

RUNNING

One of the most important pieces of equipment for a runner—of any distance—is good shoes. There has been a dramatic decrease in knee injuries for runners with good shoes.

Sprinters

Sprinters doing the 100-440-yard distance are usually the heaviest of the runners. A sprint is a performance of short duration and high intensity which requires an immediate supply of energy. This energy is provided from anaerobic (without free oxygen) sources, specifically the high energy phosphate compounds, ATP and CP, which are stored within the specific muscles activated in the sprint.

Hurdlers

Hurdlers doing the 120-yard highs and 440-yard intermediates are lighter in weight than sprinters who run comparable distances. Energy is provided from anaerobic sources, as in sprinters.

Middle-Distance Runners

Runners who cover distances of 880 yards to 6 miles are lighter in weight than hurdlers. In strenuous exercise lasting several minutes, the major source of energy comes from the anaerobic process of glycolysis with the resulting formation of lactic acid, which after a rest period is used in a reverse process of energy availability. Intense exercise of an intermediate duration performed for five to ten minutes represents a blend of metabolic energy demand. Under these conditions it is desirable to possess a high capacity for both aerobic and anaerobic metabolism.

Long-Distance Runners

Long distance runners cover six miles and above, and are the lightest weight runners of all. Due to the nature of their event, cross country runners and other endurance athletes are engaged in high levels of energy expenditure over prolonged periods of time, and will need special dietary attention. See "Carbohydrates to Glycogen" in Chapter 16 and "Exercise

Drinks" in Chapter 14. The vastly increased caloric demands of the endurance athlete should be accommodated by a balanced increase in the foods in the basic four groups. The distance runners, including those running cross country, can benefit from the alternately low and high carbohydrate intakes of carbohydrate packing. See Chapter 15 to become familiar with the problems of heat during distance running.

Performances of long duration such as marathon running require a fairly constant aerobic energy supply.

Statistical evidence indicates that typical running weight (in pounds) is approximately twice a man's height (in inches). This suggests that a 70-inch man wouldn't vary much from the 140-pound weight class.

SKIING

Cross-Country Skiing

Cross-country skiing is strenuous exercise lasting an undetermined length of time. There is need of energy from aerobic metabolism. This kind of exercise requires about sixteen calories per minute. Eating well-balanced meals is recommended with energy needs depending upon length and intensity of exercise that is undertaken.

Down-Hill Skiing

In downhill skiing, lasting several minutes, the major source of energy comes from the anaerobic process of glycolysis. Intense exercise of an intermediate duration performed for five to ten minutes represents a blend of metabolic energy demand. Under these conditions it is desirable to possess a high capacity for both anaerobic and aerobic metabolism.

SOCCER

Soccer requires overall strength in all major muscle groups. Soccer is strenuous exercise and of intermediate duration. The game is very intense, and for the spurts of energy needed, the major source comes from the anaerobic process of glycolysis. As the activity increases and time of game lengthens, there will be increased formation of lactic acid. After a sufficient rest period, this formation will be available for energy. It is a unique reversal process whereby energy is efficiently made available to the muscle cells. Because of the intensity of game play as well as length of play, it is desirable that the athlete possess a high capacity for both anaerobic and aerobic metabolism.

SWIMMING

Because there is no dust or pollen to contend with, swimming has been found to be an ideal sport for asthmatics.

Since women have a higher percentage of body fat—proportionately—than men, physiologists suggest that women's success in distance swimming results from their greater buoyancy and resistance to cold.

Swimmers depend on arms and shoulders for particular power so they will need to concentrate on their upper body development for increased strength.

Eating a good basic diet is important for swimmers. Both training and competitive performances can be enhanced by a good diet. What to eat and when to eat are particular problems for swimmers. Food before an early morning workout is not necessary, but if the swimmer wants food, orange or grapefruit juice and toast and jelly or honey would be good. When the swimmer is involved in twice a day workouts, he or she will function well on three meals—dividing the calories about equally between the three meals. If snacks are desired in addition to the regular meals, that will depend on the needs of the athlete. Many swimmers are very young and still growing, so their needs will be for various amounts of foods. Eat to satisfy the body needs, but not to become overweight. (See suggestion on pre-event eating in the beginning of Chapter 12.)

Performances of short duration and high intensity such as

the twenty-five-yard swim, require an immediate supply of energy. This energy is provided from anaerobic sources, specifically the high energy phosphate compounds, ATP and CP, stored within the particular muscles that are exercised.

In strenuous exercise lasting several minutes, the major source of energy comes from the anaerobic process of glycolysis. Intense exercise of an intermediate duration performed for five to ten minutes represents a blend of metabolic energy demands. Thus it is desirable to possess a high capacity for both anaerobic and aerobic metabolism.

Performances of long duration, such as distance swimming, require a fairly constant aerobic energy supply. Carbohydrate packing, described in Chapter 11, has proven beneficial to competitors in the middle distance and longer swim events.

Swimmers use between five to ten calories per minute, depending on speed and intensity of exercise.

TENNIS

Tennis requires overall strength in all major muscle groups. Competitive tennis is a strenuous exercise lasting several minutes, thus the major source of energy comes from the anaerobic process of glycolysis with the resulting formation of lactic acid. Rest periods between matches can help utilize the lactic acid that has been formed. Intense exercise of an intermediate duration performed for five to ten minutes represents a blend of metabolic energy demands. For long, intense action and for tournament play, it is desirable to possess a high capacity for both aerobic and anaerobic metabolism.

Tennis competition often involves long tournaments; matches may be scheduled at various times over a period of days, and many times the matches are played out of doors in hot weather—other times, indoors. Liquid consumption is critical—schedule frequent water breaks. Eat regular meals, as close to your normal eating times as possible. (See Suggestions on pre-event eating in the beginning of Chapter 12.) Supplement regular meals with sweetened drinks or hard candies, if this appeals. Omit anything that isn't needed to maintain proper electrolyte balance and necessary energy. About seven to ten calories per minute are needed in a fast game of tennis.

WEIGHT LIFTING

Weight lifting is a performance of short duration and high intensity. It requires an immediate supply of energy provided exclusively from anaerobic sources, specifically the high-energy phosphate compounds ATP and CP. This is stored within the specific muscles which are exercised and used in the weight-lifting activity.

Muscle mass and strength development programs should be supervised under diet and exercise conditions.

About eight calories per minute are required during actual weight lifting.

WRESTLING

Wrestling requires not only explosive body movements, but constant aggression against the resistance of the opponent and immediate response to his counter moves. It combines some features similar to other sports in terms of energy. It is characterized by intermittent periods of moderate activity with sudden spurts of anaerobic energy expenditure. During the anaerobic process of glycolysis there may be a resulting formation of lactic acid. Rest periods between matches (such as in tournament activity) can help utilize the lactic acid as a form of energy. A wrestler uses about four calories of energy per minute and up to three times this amount for short spurts of activity.

Excess body weight is not functional in most weight brackets, but in the heavyweight bracket, increased body mass may be advantageous.

Carbohydrate packing may be effective for a wrestler during tournament time, see Chapter 11. "Exercise Drinks" in Chapter 14; "Weight Reduction", Chapter 9; and "Eating—Pre-event, During and After," Chapter 12, can be helpful to the wrestler.

Appendix

Some Recipes to Help the Athlete

LIQUID MEAL RECIPE

½ cup non-fat dry milk
3 cups skim milk
½ cup water
¼ cup sugar
1 teaspoon flavoring (vanilla)

Add all ingredients and blend. The nutrients in liquid meals are quickly absorbed into the body. They are suggested before endurance activities or for one under stress. 1 cup will provide 100 calories. Liquid meal will leave the stomach in about 2 hours.

FRUIT MILK SHAKES

2 cups of milk
Add 1 mashed banana or
½ cup crushed sweetened strawberries, or
other berries, or
½ cup mashed sweetened peaches, or
2 cups orange juice + ¼ tsp. almond extract
Add a scoop of ice cream if you like

Shake or beat until well blended and frothy. NOTE: Use
ANY fruit you like (about ½ cup for 2 cups milk). Use ANY
fruit juice (you may want to add a little sugar).

RUSSIAN SPICE TEA MIX

½ cup powdered orange drink mix
½ cup instant tea
1 cup sugar (less if you wish)
3 tablespoons powdered lemonade mix
1 teaspoon each of cinnamon and cloves

Mix the ingredients together and use 2 teaspoons of it per cup;
fill the cup with boiling water.

HOT ORANGE DRINK

Add 1 cup hot water to 2-3 teaspoons powdered orange drink;
mix and serve hot.

HOT GELATIN DRINK

Add 3 cups boiling water to 1 package of gelatin—any flavor;
serve hot.

ORAL ELECTROLYTE SOLUTIONS (Exercise Drinks)

Vitamin C is lost in sweat. It is vital to the metabolism of glucose, and therefore is important in an exercise drink.

To any of the following, add a scant ¼ teaspoon of salt to one quart of liquid:

Orange juice (may be diluted)
Lemonade
Apple cider
Skim milk
Grapefruit juice

For an inexpensive hot weather workout drink, add 1 teaspoon of salt to 6 quarts of *flavored* water.

The exact formula of a commercial electrolyte drink is a guarded secret. If you buy an exercise drink, *READ THE LABEL . . . KNOW WHAT YOU ARE GETTING BESIDES EXPENSIVE WATER!*

HOMEMADE CHICKEN SOUP

2 quarts of water
2 chicken backs, necks, and wings
2 onions, quartered
2 carrots, quartered
2 ribs of celery, quartered
1-2 teaspoons salt
2 sprigs of parsley
Optional: 4 peppercorns
**   2 bay leaves**

Wash chicken parts. Cover with cold water and add seasonings. Bring to a boil and skim away the protein waste which forms on the surface. When the soup is cleared, add vegetables. Reduce heat to a simmer. Cover and cook for 40 minutes.

For a clear broth, strain the soup and chill. Remove fat layer on top.

For chicken-noodle soup, add noodles to broth and cook until noodles are tender. Season to taste.

Chicken soup is a good food when suffering from a cold.

HOMEMADE GRANOLA

6 cups old fashioned oatmeal (not quick)
½ cup toasted wheat germ
½ cup flaked coconut
½ cup English walnuts
½ cup cashews
⅓ cup sesame seeds
⅓ cup sunflower seeds
½ cup vegetable oil
⅓ to ½ cup honey
2 tablespoons vanilla
Optional: 1-½ cups of dried fruits may be added. Choices include: raisins, apricots, prunes, apples, dates.

Spread oats on a large cookie sheet and bake in a 350° preheated oven. After oatmeal has heated through for about 10 minutes, add walnuts, cashews, wheat germ, coconut, sesame seeds and sunflower seeds. Heat vegetable oil and honey together, then add vanilla, and pour over oatmeal, seeds, etc. mixture. Blend well. Return to oven for about 15 minutes. If adding dried fruit, add during the last five minutes of baking time. If you like chunks of granola, limit stirring of the mixture. Keeps indefinitely in refrigerator. Makes about 5 pints. Recipe may be doubled.

PEANUT BUTTER DANDIES

Put into bowl and mix:
  ½ cup peanut butter
  ½ cup honey or molasses or corn syrup
Stir in a little at a time:
  1 cup dry powdered milk

Place mixture on a sheet of waxed paper. Spread ¾ inch thick and cut into squares, or form dough into a long roll and cut it into slices, or roll into small balls.

BANANA-PEANUT TREAT

Shake 1-inch chunks of peeled bananas in a bag with chopped salted peanuts to coat with nuts.

NUTTY SNACKS

Mix equal amounts of salted peanuts and raisins for nibbling.

POPCORN WITH PEANUT BUTTER

When melting maragine to pour over hot popped corn, add a spoonful of peanut butter. It blends with the butter and gives a pleasing flavor.

MUNCHIES

2-12 oz. pkgs. chocolate chips
2-6 oz. pkgs. butterscotch chips
½ cup honey
½ cup chopped dates
½ cup yellow raisins
½ cup chopped dried apricots
½ cup shredded coconut
½ cup cashews
½ cup walnuts
½ cup wheat germ
1 cup uncooked oatmeal

Melt chips in top of double boiler: add honey, pour over remaining ingredients in large bowl, mix well. Pour into greased pans and cool. Cut or break into hand sized chunks.

NUTS AND BOLTS

1 part raisins
1 part currants
2 parts sunflower seeds
½ part nuts (almonds, cashews, filberts)
½ part dried fruit (apricots, apples)
a sprinkle of sesame seeds
a sprinkle of dried coconut

This is a mixture that you can snack on anytime. It will give you plenty of nourishment.

SPECIAL FOR NIBBLERS—
NUTRITIOUS, DELICIOUS!

To help maintain an even energy level—EAT LESS, BUT EAT MORE OFTEN!

Everyone loves snacks! Snacks fill you up and taste good, but they should do more than that. Snacks can provide needed vitamins, minerals and roughage in addition to protein and carbohydrates.

Cheeses—Enjoy a variety in cubes or slices.

Eggs—Hard cooked, deviled.

Vegetable Sticks—Carrots, celery, turnip, cucumber, cauliflower, green pepper, and cabbage (wedges). Dip in sour cream, cheese, or cottage cheese dip. Stuff celery with peanut butter.

Fruits—Fresh or canned apples, sliced and spread with peanut butter, pears, oranges, grapefruit, bananas, apricots, cantaloupe, etc.

Fruits—Dried prunes, raisins, apricots, figs, and bananas.

Crackers—Spread with peanut butter.

Cookies—Oatmeal, peanut butter, molasses, and fruit cookies.

Whole Grain or Enriched Cereals and Breads.

Nuts—All kinds. Peanuts are excellent snacks.

Seeds—Sunflower, pumpkin, etc. Also seeds mixed with nuts and raisins.

Popcorn.

Fruit Juices—Rather than a fruit drink, which is a high proportion of colored water.

Milk Drinks—Shakes, malts, etc.

Homemade Breads—Containing soy flour, wheat germ, seeds, fruit, nuts, etc.

If you are encouraging your athlete to eat—make it easy for him to get a *good* snack and hard work to get a *poor one!* If your athlete is having to restrict his eating, don't tempt him with lots of good food—keep baked goods frozen and other foods out of sight!

NOTES

**RESOURCE AGENCIES FOR NUTRITION
EDUCATION MATERIAL**

American Association for
  Health, Physical Education
  and Recreation
1201 16th St. NW
Washington, DC 20036

American Dental Association
211 East Chicago Avenue
Chicago, IL 60611

American Diabetes
  Association
18 East 48th Street
New York, NY 10017

American Dietetic
  Association
620 N. Michigan Avenue
Chicago, IL 60611

American Heart Association
44 East 23rd Street
New York, NY 10010

American Home Economics
  Association
2010 Massachusetts Avenue,
  N.W.
Washington, DC 20036

American Medical
  Association
Council on Foods and
  Nutrition
535 N. Dearborn St.
Chicago, IL 60610

The Arthritis Foundation
3400 Peachtree Road, N.E.
Atlanta, GA 30326

Food and Nutrition Board
National Research Council
National Academy of
  Sciences
2101 Constitution Avenue
Washington, DC 20418

Nutrition Foundation
Office of Education
888 17th St. N. W.
Washington, DC 20006

Society for Nutrition
 Education
2140 Shattuck Avenue
Suite 1110
Berkeley, CA 94707

Superintendent of Documents
U. S. Government Printing
 Office
Washington, DC 20402

U. S. Department of
 Agriculture
Research Service
Federal Center Building
Hyattsville, MD

U. S. Department of Health,
 Education and Welfare
Public Health Service
Food and Drug
 Administration
5600 Fishers Lane
Rockville, MD 20852

World Health Organization
United Nations Plaza
New York, NY 10017

State and Local Level

Agricultural Extension Services

State and local public health departments

State universities

County Extension Offices

State capitals; county seats

Industries

General Mills
Betty Crocker Nutrition Dept.
P. O. Box 1113
Minneapolis, MN 44550

National Dairy Council
111 North Canal Street
Chicago, IL 60606

National Livestock and Meat Board
37 S. Wabash Avenue
Chicago, IL 60603

American Institute of Baking
400 E. Ontario
Chicago, IL 60611

Proctor and Gamble
P. O. Box 599
Cincinnati, OH 45201

Quaker Oats Co.
Chicago, IL 60654

Libby, McNeill & Libby
Chicago, IL 60604

Index